Entry-Level Adolescent and Adult Sexual Assault Assessment

SANE/SAFE Forensic Learning Series

Endorsed by:

International Association of Forensic Nurses

SAINT LOUIS UNIVERSITY

STM **Learning,** Inc.

Leading Publisher of Scientific, Technical, and Medical Educational Resources
Saint Louis
www.stmlearning.com

SAINT LOUIS
UNIVERSITY

ACCREDITATION:

The book's activities have been planned and implemented in accordance with the Essential Areas and Policies of the Accreditation for Continuing Medical Education and Continuing Nursing Education through the joint providership of Saint Louis University School of Medicine, Saint Louis University School of Nursing, and STM Learning, Inc.

AMERICAN MEDICAL ASSOCIATION:

Saint Louis University School of Medicine designates this enduring material for a maximum of 3.0 *AMA PRA Category 1 Credits*™. Physicians should only claim credit commensurate with the extent of their participation in the activity.

VALIDATION OF CONTENT:

Saint Louis University School of Medicine follows the ACCME policy on Validation of Content for CME activities, which requires that:

All recommendations involving clinical medicine must be based on evidence that is accepted within the profession of medicine as adequate justification for their indications and contraindications in the care of patients.

All scientific research referred to, reported, or used in CME in support or justification of a patient care recommendation must conform to the generally accepted standards of experimental design, data collection, and analysis.

ACCREDITATION NURSING:

Saint Louis University is an approved provider of continuing nursing education by the Missouri Nurses Association, an accredited approver by the American Nurses Credentialing Center's Commission on Accreditation.

Missouri Nurses Association Provider #112-VII
This material qualifies for 3.0 Nursing Contact Hours.

DISCLOSURE POLICY:

It is the policy of Saint Louis University School of Medicine and School of Nursing to ensure balance, independence, objectivity, and scientific rigor in its continuing medical education program. Faculty and planning committee members participating in these activities are required to disclose to the audiences prior to the activity the following:

The existence of any significant financial or other relationship with the manufacturer of any commercial product or provider of any commercial service discussed.

Their intention to discuss a product that is not labeled for the use under discussion.

Their intention to discuss preliminary research data.

Saint Louis University School of Medicine and School of Nursing will review this activity's disclosures and resolve all identified conflicts of interest if applicable.

Entry-Level Adolescent and Adult Sexual Assault Assessment

SANE/SAFE Forensic Learning Series

Endorsed by:

International Association of Forensic Nurses

Diana K. Faugno, MSN, RN, CPN, SANE-A, SANE-P, DF-IAFN, FAAFS
Forensic Registered Nurse Consultant
Board of Directors EVAW International
Palm Desert, California

Rachell A. Copeland, PhC, MSN, ARNP-BC
Center for Forensic Nursing Excellence
Issaquah, Washington

Jill L. Crum, BSN, RN, SANE-A
Eisenhower Medical Center
Forensic Controller
Rancho Mirage, California

Patricia M. Speck, DNSc, APN, FNP-BC, DF-IAFN, FAAFS, FAAN
Associate Professor and Public Health Nursing Option Coordinator
University of Tennessee Health Science Center, College of Nursing
Forensic Nursing Services, LLC
Memphis, Tennessee

SAINT LOUIS UNIVERSITY

STM **Learning,** Inc.

Leading Publisher of Scientific, Technical, and Medical Educational Resources
Saint Louis
www.stmlearning.com

Publishers: Glenn E. Whaley and Marianne V. Whaley
Art Design Director: Glenn E. Whaley
Managing Editor: G.W. Graphics
Associate Editor: Kimberly E. Fletcher
Book Design/Page Layout: G.W. Graphics
Print/Production Coordinator: G.W. Graphics
Cover Design: G.W. Graphics
Color Prepress Specialist: Kevin Tucker
Acquisition Editor: Glenn E. Whaley
Developmental Editor: G.W. Graphics
Copy Editor: G.W. Graphics
Proofreader: Katie Sharp

Printed in China.

Publisher:
STM Learning, Inc.
8045 Big Bend Blvd., Suite 202, Saint Louis, Missouri 63119-2714 USA
Phone: (314)993-2728 Fax: (314)993-2281 Toll Free: (800)600-0330
http://www.stmlearning.com

Library of Congress Cataloging-in-Publication Data

Entry-level adolescent and adult sexual assault assessment : SANE/SAFE forensic learning series / Diana K. Faugno ... [et al.].
p. ; cm.
SANE/SAFE forensic learning series
Includes bibliographical references and index.
ISBN 978-1-936590-00-1 (alk. paper)
I. Faugno, Diana K., 1950- II. Title: SANE/SAFE forensic learning series.
[DNLM: 1. Nursing Diagnosis--methods--Problems and Exercises. 2. Rape--diagnosis--Problems and Exercises. 3. Adolescent. 4. Adult. 5. Forensic Nursing--methods--Problems and Exercises. 6. Nurse's Role--Problems and Exercises. 7. Rape--rehabilitation--Problems and Exercises. WY 18.2]

616.07'5076--dc23

2012011205

Contributors

Toyetta L. Beukes, RN, MSN, NP, CSANE-A, CSANE-P
Director of the Sexual Assault Response Team
San Gabriel Valley Medical Center
San Gabriel, California

Jacqueline Callari-Robinson, RN
SANE Coordinator/Director of Health Services
Wisconsin Coalition Against Sexual Assault (WCASA)
Madison, Wisconsin

Amy Carney, NP, PhD
Assistant Professor
School of Nursing
California State University, San Marcos
San Marcos, California

Kim Day, RN, FNE, SANE-A, SANE-P
SAFE Technical Assistance Coordinator
International Association of Forensic Nurses
Arnold, Maryland

Merle M. Endo, RN, SANE-A, SANE-P
Hilo, Hawaii

E. J. Ernst, DNP, MBA, APRN, FNP-BC, CEN
Lecturer
California State University, Dominguez Hills
Carson, California
Nursing Service
Geriatrics and Rehabilitative Care
Veterans Administration, Greater Los Angeles
Los Angeles, California

Janean Fossum, BSN, RN, CDDN
Forensic Nurse Consultant
Certified Developmental Disabilities Nurse
Eugene, Oregon

Shannon Liew, RN, BSN, SANE-A
SANE Coordinator
Crime Victim Services Division
Office of the Illinois Attorney General
Chicago, Illinois

Stacey A. Mitchell, DNP, MBA, RN, SANE-A, SANE-P
Director
Forensic Nursing Services
Harris County Hospital District
Houston, Texas

Claire Nelli, RN, SANE-A
CEO
Independent Forensic Services
San Diego, California

Mary Reina, RN, MSN, SANE-A, SANE-P
Forensic Services Unit (FSU) Director
Antelope Valley Hospital
Lancaster, California

Sharon M. Robison, RN, SANE-A, SANE-P, MLDI
Chief Administrative Officer
Forensic Nursing Specialties
Fort Wayne Sexual Assault Treatment Center
Fort Wayne, Indiana

The authors would like to thank the many forensic nurses who continue to care for patients affected by violence worldwide.

Diana K. Faugno, MSN, RN, CPN, SANE-A, SANE-P, DF-IAFN, FAAFS
Rachell A. Copeland, PhC, MSN, ARNP-BC
Jill L. Crum, BSN, RN, SANE-A
Patricia M. Speck, DNSc, APN, FNP-BC, DF-IAFN, FAAFS, FAAN

Foreword

After completing the basic sexual assault examiner education requirements, many health care providers face challenges maintaining current knowledge and clinical competence. There are several reasons examiners struggle:

— They have limited contact with the patient population.

— They lack access to experienced clinicians qualified to provide ongoing evaluation and peer review.

— They experience professional demands that limit the time available to maintain and improve the highly specialized skills needed to care for this patient population.

In addition, much of the literature useful for SANE/SAFE continuing education and skill building is not readily accessible to practicing examiners.

The *SANE/SAFE Forensic Learning Series* is a valuable tool that supplements teaching materials during the initial educational experience as well as beyond the basic training environment. The format and content are suited for inclusion in the curriculum of any adolescent/adult sexual assault examiner course. The design is equally useful as part of an annual competency evaluation or an independent study guide for individuals wishing to sharpen their skills.

The *Entry-Level Adolescent and Adult Sexual Assault Assessment* provides the material newly trained examiners need to become more familiar with identification and analysis of case findings. Using this book allows both new and experienced examiners an opportunity to build their skills in anatomy identification, documentation, and treatment.

As an educator of forensic nurses who care for sexually victimized patients, I am heartened to know a well-developed, peer-reviewed teaching tool is now available. Comprised of realistic, clinical scenarios, this series is designed to challenge the critical-thinking skills of both novice examiners and experienced sexual assault nurse examiners looking for a review of general practice information, anatomy, and injury. The material is also valuable for managers and supervisors seeking effective methods for objective evaluation of clinical competence in experienced examiners.

Continuing professional education is a critical aspect of ensuring competent care for this unique patient population. It is now easily accessible in the *SANE/SAFE Forensic Learning Series*. I strongly recommend this series as an essential addition to every training curriculum and forensic nursing library.

Eileen Allen, MSN, RN, FN-CSA, SANE-A, SANE-P
President (2011)
International Association of Forensic Nurses

Preface

Collectively, the authors of the *SANE/SAFE Forensic Learning Series: Adolescent and Adult Sexual Assault Assessment* have more than 70 years of forensic nursing experience. In addition to direct-care services, they provide education, training, and consultation services nationally and internationally as experts in forensic nursing practice and the evaluation and management of patients with a history of sexual assault or abuse. Like other SANE/SAFE pioneers, the authors noticed an absence of evidence for practice among the early SANE/SAFE educators. Based on existing activities, there was inference about the management of patients during the early 1990s. The published literature was comprised of primarily descriptive articles explaining the role and activities of sexual assault examiners. The language used in the literature was not standardized, and providers invented their own ways to use the descriptions to explain why an injury was present or not (eg, mounting injury). Additionally there was poor understanding about historical medical nomenclature describing a genital structure and an area (eg, labia minora [structure], fossa navicularis [area]). Consequently, published materials were inconsistent, and communities adopted and promoted their own materials.

Before the 1990s, the student population was generally inexperienced and had little collective knowledge about the variety of victim presentations in need of evaluation by a sexual assault examiner. The challenge for early educators was to confirm that interpretation and description of their findings were accurate. Also, many of the photos were taken with a 35mm camera and were of poor quality, which made attaining consensus among the experts increasingly difficult. In fact, consensus as a method to bring differing camps together was not used. That began to change in the 1990s when teachers of basic sexual assault examiner education programs shared photographs from existing cases. The process of seeking confirmation was called peer review. By attending peer-review meetings, new sexual assault examiners were able to listen to and internalize the language used by the experts to interpret similar cases in their own practices.

Despite this overall progress for sexual assault examiners, many new SANEs are unsupervised and still do not experience structured peer-review processes by expert practitioners. Criminal justice professionals put incredible pressure on examiners to report a positive or negative examination, creating a potential for the over- or undercalling or misinterpretation of findings. The authors are often consulted by attorneys and hospitals after administrators realize their programs lack checks and balances to ensure consistent, evidence-based opinions through peer review with experts. To date, the authors have reviewed hundreds of cases completed by SANE providers that have been challenged because of minimal supervision and suspected bias (eg, over- or undercalling the results). Cases suspected of bias are overwhelmingly evaluated by undergraduate nurses (eg, diploma, AD, BSN) who practice without oversight and have incorrectly identified anatomical areas or misinterpreted findings. Consistently, they fail to use the evidence-based peer-review consensus process to correct variance in their opinions. It is the standard of practice for forensic nurses to participate in peer review and quality improvement. Consequently, the authors believe that all forensic cases should receive the scrutiny of a peer-review process with experts before opinions about findings are revealed. In the meantime, the problem of incorrect identification of anatomical locations, as well as misinterpretation of findings, continues in many communities, and justice is not being served for the victim or the perpetrator.

The *SANE/SAFE Forensic Learning Series: Adolescent and Adult Sexual Assault Assessment* is designed to standardize the nomenclature for anatomy as it relates to the genital, anal, and rectal areas for new and reviewing SANEs/SAFEs; medical residents and physicians; nurse practitioners, including nurse midwives, WHNPs, PNPs, and FNPs; and nursing students. Standardization of the language of sexual assault helps create consistency among the forms developed by programs within agencies, where checklists have been demonstrated to improve objectivity. The set also will teach beginning SANE/SAFE practitioners, medical residents, and nursing students the language of evidence-based evaluative methods used when caring for adolescent and adult patients reporting a history of sexual assault and the rationale for opinions formed by health care providers. The *SANE/SAFE Forensic Learning Series: Adolescent and Adult Sexual Assault Assessment* will present adolescent or adult peer-reviewed cases that have a clear history, photographic representation, and confirmation of anatomical landmarks and injury; discussions about existing conditions and their influence; identification of injuries; evidence-based collection techniques; and treatment based on recommendations made by the Centers for Disease Control and Prevention, the World Health Organization, and local protocol. Offering this resource to new SANEs/SAFEs and resident or nursing students, as well as the reviewing practitioner needing to demonstrate competency, will fulfill the need for peer-reviewed, basic information and will contribute to continuing competence among practicing health care providers.

The SANE/SAFE should use this series for basic and continuing education; reinforcing identification of anatomy, injury, and illness or conditions; interpretation of findings; and the evidence-collection process. Since half of all sexual assault cases have no or nonspecific findings, the *SANE/SAFE Forensic Learning Series: Adolescent and Adult Sexual Assault Assessment* will focus on correct anatomical terms, evaluation, and treatment as well as evidence collection from normal and injured anogenital structures. It is the authors' hope that you will find the *SANE/SAFE Forensic Learning Series: Adolescent and Adult Sexual Assault Assessment* helpful to you, your practice, and Sexual Assault Response/Resource Team programs.

Diana K. Faugno, MSN, RN, CPN, SANE-A, SANE-P, DF-IAFN, FAAFS
Rachell A. Copeland, PhC, MSN, ARNP-BC
Jill L. Crum, BSN, RN, SANE-A
Patricia M. Speck, DNSc, APN, FNP-BC, DF-IAFN, FAAFS, FAAN

Introduction

With entry-level, intermediate, and advanced components, the *SANE/SAFE Forensic Learning Series* appeals to students new to SANE/SAFE practice as well as longtime SANE/SAFE examiners seeking to hone their skills. Formatted for self-study and group instruction, the books allow for portable, straightforward learning. Each exercise and corresponding answer key is purposefully designed for a broad audience to reflect the diversity and scope of practice of sexual assault examiners. Medical professionals have the opportunity to earn continuing medical education (CME) credits or continuing nursing education (CNE) contact hours through successful completion of this book. Successful completion consists of reading the text in its entirety and filling out the chapter activities, posttests, credits/contact hours form, and evaluation form. The *SANE/SAFE Forensic Learning Series* is a valuable resource to trainees, early stage practitioners, and managers and supervisors responsible for the ongoing evaluation of examiners.

Self-Study Use

Using case studies and attendant color photographs, the *SANE/SAFE Forensic Learning Series* simulates the environment of a clinic.

The *Entry-Level Adolescent and Adult Sexual Assault Assessment* is the first in a series of books that provides continuing education to examiners who assess and treat patients reporting a history of sexual assault or abuse.

Group Instructional Use

The *Entry-Level Adolescent and Adult Sexual Assault Assessment* provides instructors with the materials they need to share knowledge of sexual assault and abuse issues with interested participants. Approval to teach this material for CME credits or CNE contact hours must be obtained through the appropriate channels. Please refer to the section titled "Teaching a Class for CME Credits/CNE Contact Hours" on page xv.

Students should purchase their own copies of the *Entry-Level Adolescent and Adult Sexual Assault Assessment* when learning in a classroom setting. The registration number printed on the inside cover of the book is required to apply for CME credits or CNE contact hours. Students should register and pay for CME credits or CNE contact hours as outlined in the section titled "Obtaining Continuing Education Certificate of Completion" on page xiv.

Use for Medical Professionals

Professionals seeking CME credits or CNE contact hours can obtain them through the successful completion of this book. Three CME credits or CNE contact hours can be earned.

SANE/SAFE Forensic Learning Series
Offering Lifelong Learning for Medical Professionals

The best training for the best medical professionals

Authors:
Diana K. Faugno, MSN, RN, CPN, SANE-A, SANE-P, DF-IAFN, FAAFS
Rachell A. Copeland, PhC, MSN, ARNP-BC
Jill L. Crum, BSN, RN, SANE-A
Patricia M. Speck, DNSc, APN, FNP-BC, DF-IAFN, FAAFS, FAAN

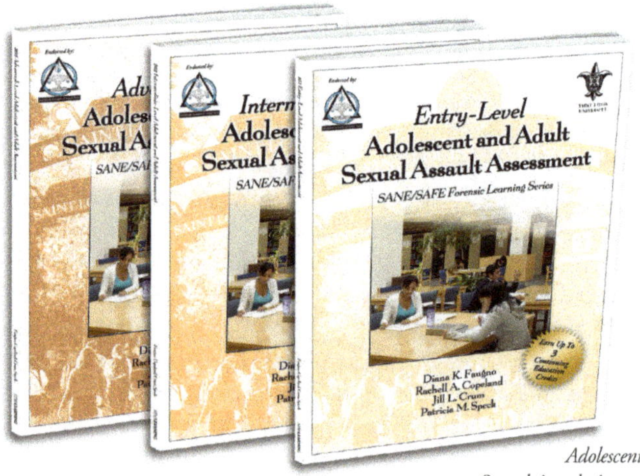

Adolescent and Adult Sexual Assault Assessment Shown

SAINT LOUIS UNIVERSITY

The book's activities have been planned and implemented in accordance with the Essential Areas and Policies of the Accreditation for Continuing Medical Education and Continuing Nursing Education through the joint providership of Saint Louis University School of Medicine, Saint Louis University School of Nursing, and STM Learning, Inc.

SANE/SAFE Forensic Learning Series

An Overview

STM Learning's ***SANE/SAFE Forensic Learning Series: Adolescent and Adult Sexual Assault Assessment*** is designed to challenge the critical thinking skills of sexual assault examiners responsible for identifying injuries, collecting evidence, and treating patients reporting a history of sexual assault or abuse.

This highly anticipated series gives students an opportunity to learn, apply, and demonstrate competency in sexual assault evaluations of adolescents and adults. The Entry-Level, Intermediate-Level, and Advanced-Level books include an anatomical review for oral, genital, and anal anatomy; case studies with identification, documentation, and treatment activities; comprehensive answer keys; and questions that test the comprehension of overall content.

Materials and activities in the ***SANE/SAFE Forensic Learning Series*** have been accredited through the Saint Louis University School of Medicine and the Saint Louis University School of Nursing. Medical professionals can earn 3.0 AMA PRA Category 1 Credits™ or 3.0 Nursing Contact Hours.

Features and Benefits

— Accredited through the Saint Louis University School of Medicine and the Saint Louis University School of Nursing for 3.0 AMA PRA Category 1 Credits™ or 3.0 Nursing Contact Hours
— Authored by internationally known SANE/SAFE experts
— Endorsed by the International Association of Forensic Nurses
— Formatted for self-study and group instruction
— Written for a broad audience to capture the diversity and scope of practice of sexual assault examiners
— Portable size and affordable price

Order by phone 314-993-2728 or online www.stmlearning.com.

Instructions

Overview

The *SANE/SAFE Forensic Learning Series* was developed to be used in conjunction with, or after, an official SANE training course that meets the International Association of Forensic Nurses Educational Guidelines.

Application of clinical reasoning is hard for all learners. The authors of this book believe that repetition improves deconstruction of the relevant educational information needed in critical thinking, but more importantly, it improves the clinical reasoning necessary for quality evidenced-based practice. In the *SANE/SAFE Forensic Learning Series*, participants will read and analyze many cases and their unique components and then critically think about the most appropriate application of clinical reasoning based on the patient history, identification of anatomical locations, and specific injury, whether intentional or unintentional. These cases focus on evaluation and documentation from case histories and physical findings, but with each book in the series, cases include increasingly complex social situations that present in many SANE/SAFE programs. The authors assume the SANE/SAFE provider has collected or demonstrates collection of a locally approved Sexual Assault Examination Kit. Throughout the *SANE/SAFE Forensic Learning Series*, peer-reviewed answers reflect the students' efforts to gather knowledge from a variety of areas to achieve clinical reasoning about each case study, including what, if any, additional evidence should be collected and which medical treatment interventions are necessary. For instance, what should be collected if the patient shaves his or her external genital area or was grabbed forcefully? A basic premise for the *SANE/SAFE Forensic Learning Series* is that providers learn by doing and through repetition that includes the use of correct anatomical descriptions, injury identification, and medical treatment. With repetition, the SANE/SAFE will master the knowledge, skills, abilities, and understanding required for a quality, peer-reviewed practice.

Educational Objectives

At the conclusion of this book, students will be able to:

— Locate and describe structures of the oral, genital, and anal anatomy for adolescent and adult patients reporting a history of sexual assault.

— List recommendations for preventing and treating sexually transmitted infections as recommended by the Centers for Disease Control and Prevention, the World Health Organization, and the student's local protocol.

— Identify injuries to the oral, genital, and anal anatomy for adolescent and adult patients reporting a history of sexual assault.

— Document oral, genital, and anal injuries in adolescent and adult patients reporting a history of sexual assault.

— List items to be collected for evidentiary purposes for adolescent and adult patients reporting a history of sexual assault.

— Use standard terminology for documenting the medical forensic evaluation, including photodocumentation.

— Use standard terminology for describing items collected for evidentiary purposes, including photodocumentation.

— Define drug-facilitated sexual assault and describe the evidence to be collected.

— Demonstrate use of photodocumentation in case reviews of adolescent and adult patients reporting a history of sexual assault.

Expected Outcomes

The *SANE/SAFE Forensic Learning Series* provides continuing education to forensic nurses who assess and treat patients reporting a history of sexual assault or abuse. Physicians and physicians' assistants will qualify for *AMA PRA Category 1 Credit*™ and nurses will qualify for ANA continuing education contact hours.

Course Format and Implementation

For optimal results, we suggest you read the text in its entirety and complete the chapter activities and posttests. The entire course takes 2 to 3 hours to complete.

Chapters and credits designated for this book are as follows:

Chapter 1 – Sexual Assault: 41-year-old Female Patient with Down's Syndrome

Chapter 2 – Sexual Assault: 32-year-old Male Patient

Chapter 3 – Incapacitated Sexual Assault: 24-year-old Female Patient

Chapter 4 – Sexual Assault: 21-year-old Female College Student

Chapter 5 – Drug-Facilitated Sexual Assault: 15-year-old Female Patient

Chapter 6 – Sexual Assault: 17-year-old Female Patient

Chapter 7 – Incapacitated Sexual Assault: 24-year-old Female Patient in a Psychiatric Facility

Chapter 8 – Sexual Assault and Intimate Partner Violence: 32-year-old Female Patient

Chapter 9 – Sexual Assault: 20-year-old Female Patient

Chapter 10 – Documenting a History and Reviewing a Case

Total: 3.0 credits

Obtaining Continuing Education Certificate of Completion

Physicians, physicians' assistants, and nurses wishing to obtain CME credits or CNE contact hours must complete and return the posttest, credits/contact hours form, and evaluation form for the book for which they are seeking credit. Posttests with a score of 80 percent or better will be considered passing. Participants will be awarded a certificate of completion for the completed book purchased for CME credits or CNE contact hours. In order to receive your completion certificate, the posttest, credits/contact hours form, and evaluation form must be filled out completely and returned to the appropriate department at Saint Louis University.

All documents required to receive American Medical Association (AMA) certificate of completion can be accessed through the Saint Louis University CME website. Please visit: http://www.slu.edu/x54431.xml. Once the site has loaded, click the title and ISBN number that matches the book you have completed and follow the online instructions. If you are unable to submit all required forms through the Saint Louis University CME website, photocopy the posttest, evaluation form, and credits/contact hours form; complete; and return by post or electronic mail. The book registration number must be written on all forms to receive CME credits or CNE contact hours. The registration number can be used only once and is printed on the inside front cover of this book.

Participants will be assessed a fee for each certificate of completion issued. Certificates are available for $45 for CME or $25 for CNE participants. Payment must accompany the return of the posttest and evaluation form. Acceptable methods of payment are money order, personal check, and credit/debit card. Please make all checks payable to Saint Louis University.

SUBMIT BY DIGITAL FORM:
Website address: http://www.slu.edu/x54431.xml

SUBMIT BY POST OR ELECTRONIC MAIL:

For CME: Saint Louis University School of Medicine
Program Director, Continuing Medical Education
Saint Louis University – Young Hall
3839 Lindell Boulevard
St. Louis, MO 63108
314-977-7401
cme@slu.edu

For CNE: Saint Louis University School of Nursing
Coordinator of Continuing Nursing Education
Saint Louis University
3525 Caroline Mall
St. Louis, MO 63104
314-977-8919

You will receive the certificate of completion within 4 weeks after receipt of your test and evaluation form. In the event you fail the test, you will be notified regarding a retake examination of the same concepts. Participants can attempt to pass each test no more than 3 times.

Physicians Only

Rush processing of your certificate is available. An additional processing fee of $25 applies. You must contact the Saint Louis University Continuing Medical Education office at (314) 977-7401 for application instructions. Your request will be processed and a certificate will be e-mailed to the address provided during registration within 3 to 4 business days after receipt of your test (pending pass/fail results). Mail requests do not qualify for rush processing.

Teaching a Class for CME Credits/CNE Contact Hours

If you wish to teach a class and have participants receive CME credits or CNE contact hours for attending, please contact the appropriate department at Saint Louis University.

For CME: Saint Louis University School of Medicine
Program Director, Continuing Medical Education
Saint Louis University – Young Hall
3839 Lindell Boulevard
St. Louis, MO 63108
314-977-7401
cme@slu.edu

For CNE: Saint Louis University School of Nursing
Coordinator of Continuing Nursing Education
Saint Louis University
3525 Caroline Mall
St. Louis, MO 63104
314-977-8919

Approved instructors should suggest each student purchase his or her own copy of the book when learning in a classroom setting. The registration number printed on the inside cover of the book will be required to apply for CME credits or CNE contact hours. Participants of the class will register and pay for CME credits or CNE contact hours as outlined in the section titled "Obtaining Continuing Education Certificate of Completion" (page xiv).

Accreditation Material

Saint Louis University School of Nursing

Saint Louis University School of Nursing is an approved provider of continuing nursing education by the Missouri Nurses Association, an accredited approver by the American Nurses Credentialing Center's Commission on Accreditation.

Missouri Nurses Association Provider #112-VII.

Saint Louis University School of Medicine Essential Mission Statement

The essential mission of the Continuing Medical Education program at Saint Louis University School of Medicine is to facilitate educational activities that maintain and increase the knowledge, technical skill, and competence of the practicing physician to deliver optimal health care consistent with the mission of the School of Medicine and the University. This includes, but is not limited to: updating knowledge and technical skills, providing clinical and practice management instruction, defining the functions of various health professionals and the role of the interdisciplinary team, certifying/affirming basic and advanced medical skills, and developing appropriate physician-patient relationships. The Continuing Medical Education program at Saint Louis University School of Medicine strives to initiate and encourage lifelong learning habits in its graduate, postgraduate, faculty, and community physicians.

Accreditation

This activity has been planned and implemented in accordance with the Essential Areas and Policies of the Accreditation Council for Continuing Medical Education through the joint providership of Saint Louis University School of Medicine, Saint Louis University School of Nursing, and STM Learning, Inc.

Saint Louis University School of Medicine is accredited by the Accreditation Council for Continuing Medical Education (ACCME) to provide continuing medical education for physicians.

American Medical Association

Saint Louis University School of Medicine designates this enduring material for a maximum of 3.0 *AMA PRA Category 1 Credits*™.

Physicians should only claim credit commensurate with the extent of their participation in the activity.

Validation of Content

Saint Louis University School of Medicine follows the ACCME policy on Validation of Content for CME activities, which requires that:

—All recommendations involving clinical medicine must be based on evidence that is accepted within the profession of medicine as adequate justification for their indications and contraindications in the care of patients.

—All scientific research referred to, reported, or used in CME in support or justification of a patient care recommendation must conform to the generally accepted standards of experimental design, data collection, and analysis.

Disclosure Policy

It is the policy of Saint Louis University School of Medicine to ensure balance, independence, objectivity, and scientific rigor in its continuing medical education program. Faculty and planning committee members participating in these activities are required to disclose to the audiences prior to the activity the following:

1. The existence of any significant financial or other relationship with the manufacturer of any commercial product or provider of any commercial service discussed.
2. Their intention to discuss a product that is not labeled for the use under discussion.
3. Their intention to discuss preliminary research data.

Saint Louis University School of Medicine will review this enduring activity's disclosures and resolve all identified conflicts of interest if applicable.

Faculty Disclosures

Saint Louis University School of Medicine has collected and reviewed the disclosure statements of the authors and contributors for this educational series and has determined that none of them disclosed any relevant financial relationships.

Saint Louis University School of Medicine has reviewed this activity's disclosures and resolved all identifiable conflicts of interest, if applicable.

Sexual Assault 2-Volume Set is the most comprehensive resource on sexual victimization!

Sexual Assault

Sexual Assault: Victimization Across the Life Span is an essential 2-volume set for professionals who may come into contact with someone who has been sexually assaulted. Professionals will find critical information on how to perform a physical exam, properly document the patient's history, collect forensic evidence (including DNA analysis), and address legal and prosecution issues. *Sexual Assault: Victimization Across the Life Span* examines the theory and practice of working with sexually abused or assaulted individuals. Also, the volumes help physicians to recognize the different experiences and presentations of adults and children, providing specific approaches to each. Individual sections are devoted to the unique problems of sexual victimization for children, adolescents, and adults. Other invaluable chapters on domestic violence, acquaintance rape, male sexual assault, sexual assault in correctional settings, assault of the elderly, and victimization of people with disabilities are included.

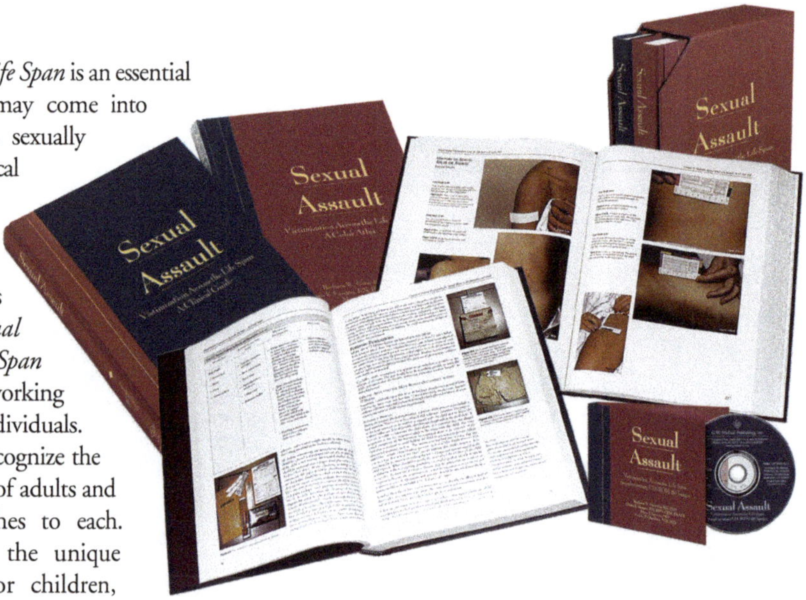

Sexual Assault

A Clinical Guide, Color Atlas, and Supplementary CD-ROM

Angelo P. Giardino, MD, PhD; Elizabeth M. Datner, MD; Janice B. Asher, MD; Barbara W. Girardin, RN, PhD; Diana K. Faugno, RN, BSN, CPN, FAAFS, SANE-A; Mary J. Spencer, MD

1435 pages, 1830 images, with 69 contributors

Sexual Assault and Supplementary CD-ROM *ISBN 978-1-878060-47-1* **$326.00**

Sexual Assault Quick Reference

Sexual Assault Quick Reference highlights assault and nonassault findings to aid in the formation of a diagnosis. Topics unique to the sexual victimization of children, adolescents, and adults are presented. Other valuable information on domestic violence, acquaintance rape, male sexual assault, sexual assault in correctional settings, assault of the elderly, and victimization of people with disabilities is included. In addition, guidelines for providing much-needed emotional and social support are addressed, including the involvement of mental health and other practitioners. Difficulties and special concerns faced by parents are also touched upon.

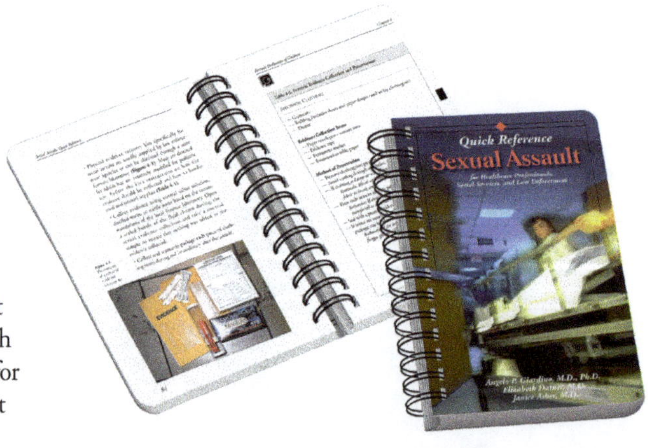

Sexual Assault Quick Reference

For Healthcare, Social Service, and Law Enforcement Professionals

Angelo P. Giardino, MD, PhD; Elizabeth M. Datner, MD; Janice B. Asher, MD; Barbara W. Girardin, RN, PhD; Diana K. Faugno, RN, BSN, CPN, FAAFS, SANE-A; Mary J. Spencer, MD

576 pages, 163 images, with 69 contributors

Sexual Assault Quick Reference *ISBN 978-1-878060-38-9* **$55.00**

Order by phone 314-993-2728 or online www.stmlearning.com.

CME Credit/CNE Contact Hours Form

Date: ____________________

If you are unable to submit all required forms through the Saint Louis University CME website, photocopy the posttest, evaluation form, and credits/contact hours form; complete; and return by post or electronic mail. (Please print.)

ISBN #: 978-1-936590-00-1

Registration number (located on inside front cover): ____________________________

Date of birth: ____________________________

Send the certificate to:
Name: ____

Title: ____________________________ Specialty: ____________________________

Company/Organization: ____

Address: ____

City/State/Zip: ____

Phone: ( ) ____________________________ Fax: ( ) ____________________________

E-mail address: ____

Please indicate how you would prefer your name to appear on the certificate. (Please print.)

____

Method of payment:
Credit Card __ Visa __ MasterCard

Cardholder's Name: ____

Card Number: __ __ __ __ - __ __ __ __ - __ __ __ __ - __ __ __ __

Expiration Date: _____ / _____ CVV Code: __ __ __

Signature of Cardholder: ______________________________________

___ Check enclosed in U.S. funds (Make payable to Saint Louis University.)

Please send your completed forms and payment to:

For CME:

Saint Louis University School of Medicine
Program Director, Continuing Medical Education
Saint Louis University – Young Hall
3839 Lindell Boulevard
St. Louis, MO 63108
314-977-7401
cme@slu.edu

For CNE:

Saint Louis University School of Nursing
Coordinator of Continuing Nursing Education
Saint Louis University
3525 Caroline Mall
St. Louis, MO 63104
314-977-8919

If you have any questions about receiving CME credit, call (314) 977-7401; questions about CNE contact hours, call (314) 977-8919.

Evaluation Form

Date: ____________________

If you are unable to submit all required forms through the Saint Louis University CME website, photocopy the posttest, evaluation form, and credits/contact hours form; complete; and return by post or electronic mail.

After finishing the course, please take a few minutes to respond to these questions. If you are applying for CME credits or CNE contact hours, a certificate of completion will not be issued until the posttest and evaluation form are returned.

ISBN #: 978-1-936590-00-1

Registration number (located on inside front cover): ____________________________

Name: __________________________________

Title: ___________________________________ Specialty: ________________________________

Date of birth: _________________________

Rate your answers to the following statements on a scale of 1 to 5.

1=Strongly Agree 2=Agree 3=Undecided 4=Disagree 5=Strongly Disagree

1. The course was well organized. ___
2. Learning objectives and assignments were clear. ___
3. The lessons were practical and applicable to actual situations. ___
4. The activities fit well within the time allotted. ___
5. I will be able to put the information learned into practice. ___
6. This course encouraged me to think. ___
7. I would recommend this course to others in my field. ___

Briefly answer the following questions.

1. What suggestions would you make to improve this course?

2. Was the content biased in any way? If yes, please explain.

3. May we contact you in 3 months with a short questionnaire to gauge the effectiveness of the program? Please list how you would prefer to be contacted.

If you have any questions about receiving CME credit, call (314) 977-7401; questions about CNE contact hours, call (314) 977-8919.

Evaluation form for Entry-Level Adolescent and Adult Sexual Assault Assessment ISBN: 978-1-936590-00-1

Reviews

The distinguished authors of the Entry-Level Adolescent and Adult Sexual Assault Assessment *provide entry-level forensic practitioners with a comprehensive resource that defines explicit circumstances related to caring for the sexually assaulted patient. The book uses photographs and an anatomical review to engage the forensic care provider, includes detailed case studies and injury identification exercises, and concludes with activities involving documentation and implementation. These activities emulate the nursing process brilliantly and encourage further reading to advance to a superior level of care.*

Jane A. Reynolds, BSN, RN, FN, CSA, SANE-P
SANE/SART Coordinator
Mercer County SANE/SART Program
Trenton, New Jersey

Using the Entry-Level Adolescent and Adult Sexual Assault Assessment *as a resource for new SANEs will enhance their ability to develop critical-thinking skills as they work through different case scenarios. The case presentations are succinct and thorough, and the photographs are excellent. The questions are structured to help develop the learner's ability to recognize basic anatomical genital structures, identify injury and what evidence should be collected, and develop a plan of care for the patient, including medications. Completing this book will make new forensic nurses feel more confident as they develop their own expertise.*

Cynthia Cook, RN, BS, SANE-A
SAFE Coordinator
Community SAFE Team
Boise, Idaho

In the Entry-Level Adolescent and Adult Sexual Assault Assessment, *the Contents in Detail provide the reader with a well-defined outline of the chapter and activities to be implemented as they relate to specifics of the sexual assault case. The sequential order of anatomical locations, injury identification, evidence collection, and treatment teaches the exam protocol. The case aids the reader or SANE with specifics of other disorders that may present with the victim in addition to the assault. The comprehensiveness of the chapter provides the reader or SANE the knowledge and skill set to conduct a thorough medical-legal sexual assault examination.*

Olga Craine-Carmichael, BSN, RN, MA
Forensic Nurse Examiner
SANE-A, SANE-C/A, SANE-C/P
Domestic Violence Specialist
North Texas Child Advocacy Center
Dallas, Texas

The Entry-Level Adolescent and Adult Sexual Assault Assessment *is going to be a "must have" addition to the forensic nursing education "tool kit" for not only practicing examiners, but forensic educators as well. The content outlines the most common case examples that examiners will encounter in their clinical work. The case studies will test the entry-level skills of examiners, thus enabling practitioners to increase their skill and knowledge in "real life" scenarios.*

For the educator, the book provides examples that can be used in a variety of venues including basic education, continuing education, and multidisciplinary discussions.

Sheila Early RN, BScN, SANE-A
Coordinator/Instructor
Forensic Health Sciences Option
Forensic Science and Technology
British Columbia Institute of Technology
Burnaby, British Columbia, Canada

The authors of the Entry-Level Adolescent and Adult Sexual Assault Assessment *have provided a valuable resource for entry-level forensic nurses, as well as advance-practice forensic nurses working in the specialty area of sexual assault and sexual abuse. The book provides a demonstration of the various types of case scenarios that forensic nurses will encounter in their practice of sexual assault. The expert knowledge base presented in this book is excellent. This resource provides forensic nurses with a challenge to improve their use of critical thinking, encouraging them to seek more education in the field of sexual assault. The use of this resource from the experts in this specialty area will aid forensic nurses in the development and improvement of their clinical performance when dealing with sexual assault survivors. This resource will aid nurses in improving the care for better patient outcomes in their nursing practice.*

Caroline Long, RN, BSN, CNOR, SANE-A
Registered Nurse
Intensive Care at St. Joseph's Hospital
Buckhannon, West Virginia
Mobile Regional SANE Team
United Hospital Center
Clarksburg, West Virginia

Contents in Brief

Contents in Detail

Entry-Level Adolescent and Adult Sexual Assault Assessment

SANE/SAFE Forensic Learning Series

Endorsed by:

International Association of Forensic Nurses

SAINT LOUIS UNIVERSITY

STM **Learning,** Inc.

Leading Publisher of Scientific, Technical, and Medical Educational Resources

Saint Louis

www.stmlearning.com

Anatomical Review

Objectives

After reviewing the figures presented in this section, the student will be able to:

1. *Correctly identify oral, genital, and anal anatomy.*
2. *Accurately define structures of the oral, genital, and anal anatomy.*

Instructions

Anatomical diagrams and photographs have been provided to assist the student with correctly identifying anatomical landmarks. These diagrams and photos should be used when documenting normal anatomy, injuries, and any other variant conditions or findings throughout the *Entry-Level Adolescent and Adult Sexual Assault Assessment.*

Additional Definitions

The student may find reviewing the following definitions useful in completing the activities within this book. Terminology for indicators of direction when documenting findings during a medical forensic examinaion include anterior, posterior, inferior, superior, medical, lateral, proximal, and distal.

— ***Abrasions:*** Superficial injuries representing the removal of the outermost layers of the skin; usually caused by lateral rubbing, sliding, or compressive forces.

— ***Avulsion:*** A forceful separation or detachment that may occur traumatically or surgically; tearing away of a body part or structure.

— ***Bruises*** (contusions): Injuries that lie below the intact epidermis and result from extravascular collection of blood that has leaked from ruptured capillaries or blood vessels after sufficient force has been applied to distort the soft tissues and tear one or more vessels.

— ***Cut:*** An opening in the skin that occurs when a sharp object comes into contact with skin or tissue with enough pressure to divide it; cuts have even, regular edges.

— ***Drug-facilitated sexual assault*** (DFSA): Generic term for all types of sexual assault when drugs, alcohol, or other intoxicants are deliberately given to the victim by the perpetrator.

— ***Lacerations:*** Injuries that occur when the continuity of the skin is broken and disrupted by blunt force such as tearing, ripping, crushing, overstretching, pulling apart, over-bending, or shearing of tissue.

— ***Incapacitated rape:*** Self-induced intoxication creating self-vulnerability and lack of consent prior to rape.

— ***Petechiae:*** Multiple hemorrhagic spots, pinpoint to pinhead in size.

Oral Cavity

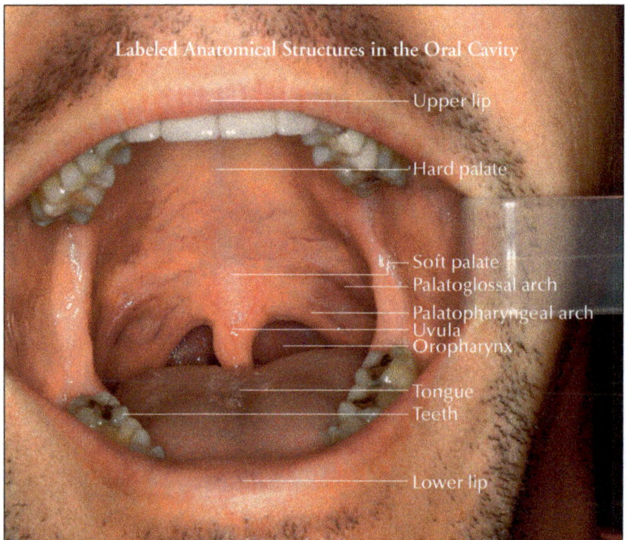

Figure AR-1

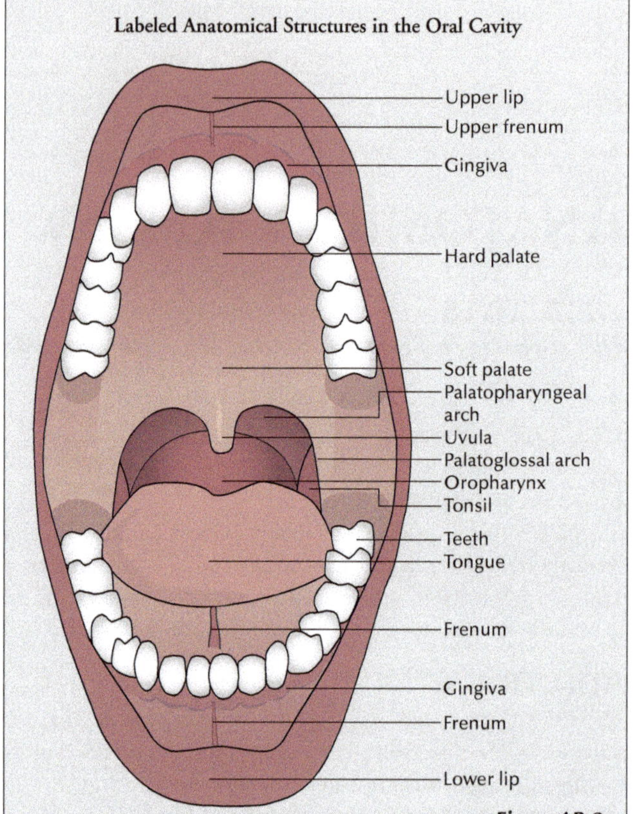

Figure AR-2

Definitions

— ***Frenum*** (original term: frenulum): A small fold of mucous membrane that limits the movements of an organ or anatomical structure (eg, lingual frenum, maxillary labial frenum, mandibular labial frenum).

— ***Gingiva:*** The soft tissue overlying the crowns of unerupted teeth and encircling the necks of those that have erupted. Wisdom teeth are the last set of molars to erupt, usually at age 18 to 25 years.

— ***Hard palate:*** The anterior part of the palate, covered above by the mucous membrane of the nose and below by the mucoperiosteum of the roof of the mouth.

— ***Lips:*** The soft external structures that form the boundaries of the mouth, the opening to the oral cavity.

— ***Oropharynx:*** The area of the pharynx between the soft palate and the upper aspect of the epiglottis; area of the throat in the back of the mouth.

— ***Palatoglossal arch:*** The anterior of the 2 folds of mucous membrane on either side of the oropharynx, enclosing the palatoglossal muscle.

— ***Palatopharyngeal arch:*** The posterior of the 2 folds of mucous membrane on either side of the oropharynx, enclosing the palatopharyngeal muscle.

— ***Soft palate:*** A movable fold consisting of muscular fibers enclosed in mucous membrane. The soft palate is suspended from the rear of the hard palate and separates the nasal cavity from the oral cavity during swallowing or sucking.

— ***Teeth:*** The hardest bone in the body. Deciduous teeth are commonly called baby teeth or primary teeth; the first set usually consists of 20 teeth. For most, there are a total of 32 permanent, or adult, teeth.

— ***Tongue:*** A mobile mass of muscular tissue that is covered with mucous membrane; occupies much of the cavity of the mouth; forms part of its floor; is the organ of taste; and assists in chewing, swallowing, and speech.

— ***Tonsil:*** A small oral mass of lymphoid tissue, especially either of 2 such masses embedded in the lateral walls of the opening between the mouth and the pharynx; it is of uncertain function, but believed to help protect the body from respiratory infections. Also called faucial tonsil or palatine tonsil.

— ***Uvula:*** A small, soft structure hanging from the free edge of the soft palate in the midline above the root of the tongue. The uvula is composed of muscle, connective tissue, and mucous membrane.

Male Genitalia

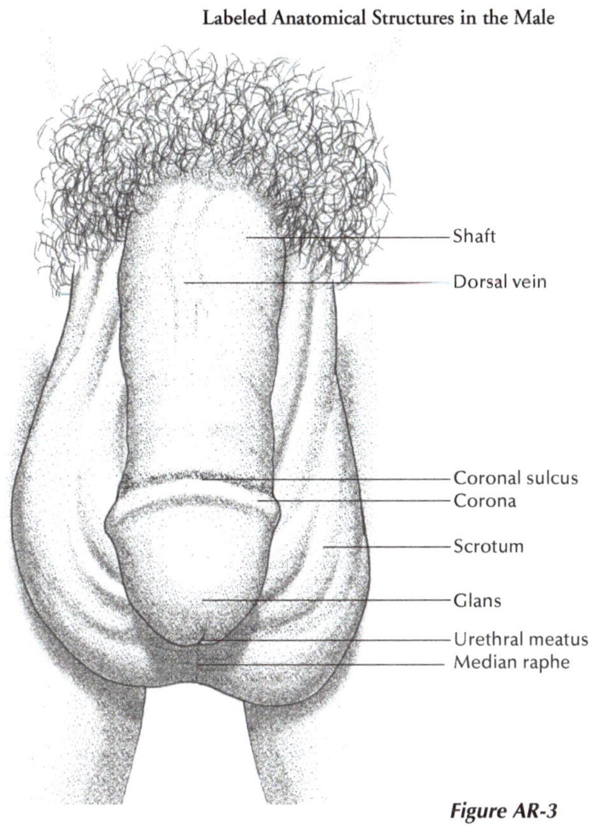

Figure AR-3

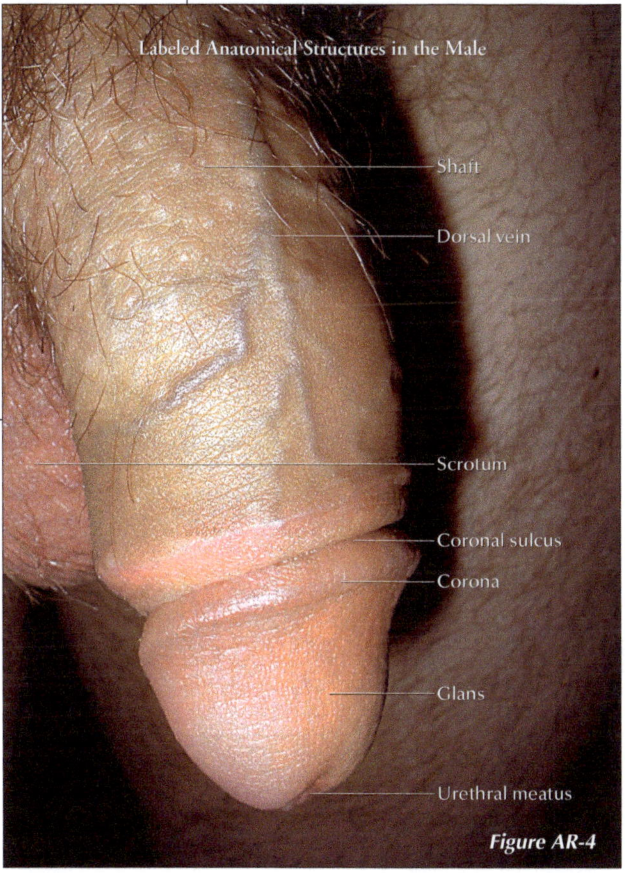

Figure AR-4

Definitions

— ***Corona of glans penis:*** The rounded, prominent border of the glans on the distal portion of the penile shaft.

— ***Coronal sulcus:*** The rounded border of the glans penis, separated from the corpora cavernosa penis by the neck of the glans.

— ***Dorsal vein:*** Tributaries spanning the dorsal surface of the penile shaft.

— ***Glans*** (also called glans penis or balanus): The cap-shaped expansion of corpus spongiosum at the distal end of the penis, which is covered by loose skin (foreskin or prepuce), enabling it to expand during an erection.

— ***Median raphe:*** A visible line of tissue extending from the anus to the perineum. The median raphe is located between the scrotum and the anus in the male and the vestibule and the anus in the female.

— ***Perineum:*** The external surface or base of the perineal body, lying between the scrotum and anus. This network of muscles, located between and around the scrotum and anus, supports the pelvic cavity and maintains the structure of the pelvic floor by keeping the organs in place.

— ***Scrotum:*** The pouch containing the testicles and their accessory organs. The scrotum is located inferiorly to the penis and is covered with hair in males of reproductive age.

— ***Shaft:*** The part of the penis between the glans and the body.

— ***Urethral meatus:*** A slit-like opening located at the tip of the glans. Urine and seminal products, including spermatozoa, exit the body through the urethral meatus.

FEMALE GENITALIA

Labeled Anatomical Structures in the Female

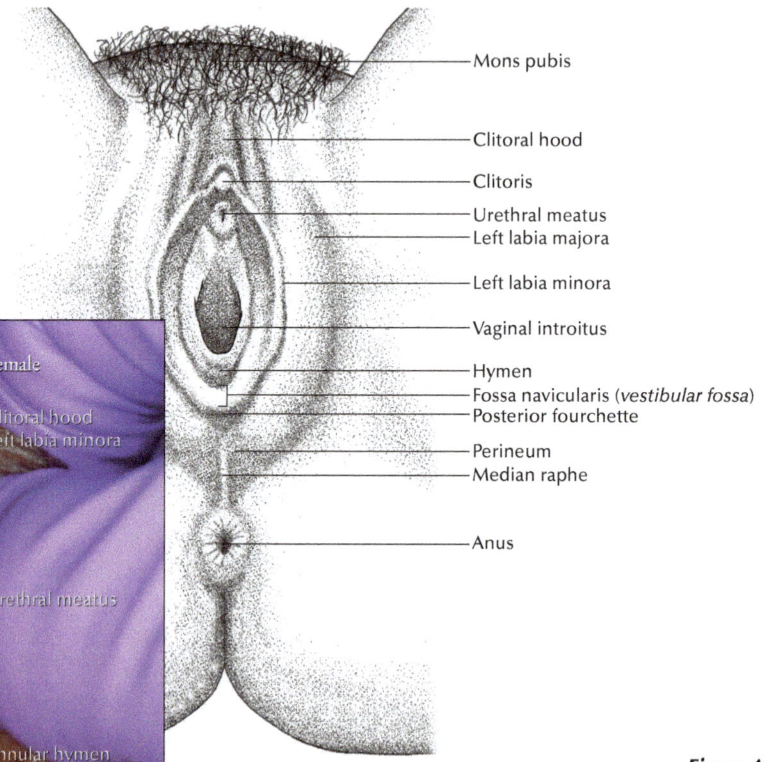

Figure AR-6

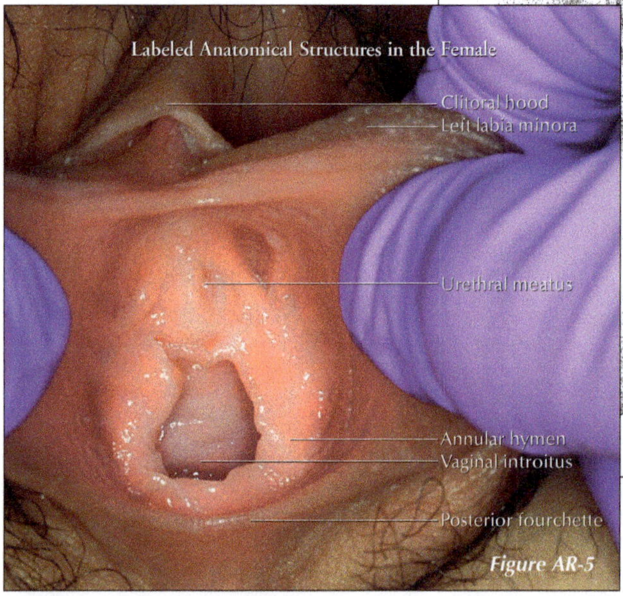

Figure AR-5

DEFINITIONS

— ***Cervical os:*** The opening in the cervix that leads to the endometrial cavity of the uterus. This area consists of unstratified columnar epithelium cells.

— ***Cervix:*** The portion of the uterus between the isthmus and the vagina.

— ***Clitoral hood:*** A fold of skin covering the clitoris.

— ***Clitoris:*** A small, cylindrical erectile body at the anterior portion of the vulva, covered by the clitoral hood.

— ***Fossa navicularis:*** The concavity of the lower part of the vestibule, posterior and inferior to the hymen corona.

— ***Hymen:*** A collar or semicollar of tissue surrounding the vaginal orifice.

— ***Labia majora:*** Two folds of skin on either side of the labia minora. This area usually is covered with hair that appears during puberty.

— ***Labia minora:*** The longitudinal thin folds of non-keratinized skin medial to the labia majora. The labia minora are hairless but have many sensory nerve endings that engorge when stimulated.

— ***Median raphe:*** A visible line of tissue extending from the anus to the perineum. It is located between the vestibule and the anus in the female and the scrotum and the anus in the male.

— ***Mons pubis:*** The rounded fleshy prominence created by adipose tissue overlying the pubic symphysis bone.

— ***Perineum:*** The external surface or base of the perineal body, lying between the vulva and anus. This network of muscles, located between and around the vagina and anus, supports the pelvic cavity and maintains the structure of the pelvic floor by keeping the organs in place.

— ***Periurethral bands*** (also called vestibular bands or urethral ligaments): Structures that support the urethra and the pelvic floor and are often confused with adhesive scarring. When seen, these bands are usually symmetrical, found in pairs, and attached to the pubic symphysis area.

— ***Posterior fornix:*** Vault-like recess inferior to the cervix; it is created from the protrusion of the cervix into the upper vagina.

— ***Posterior fourchette*** (also called Hart's line or the posterior commissure): An area where the two labia meet posteriorly.

— ***Rugae:*** Normal folds of epithelium that run circumferentially from the vaginal columns in the vagina. They are not present when there is no estrogen or estrogen effect.

SPECULUM EXAMINATION

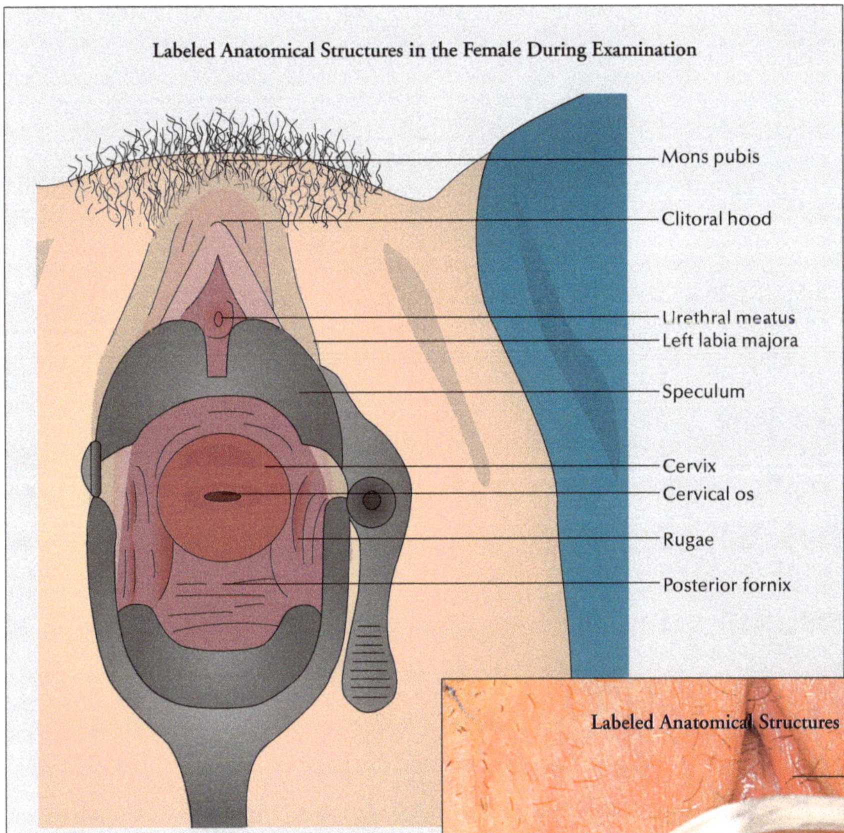

Figure AR-7

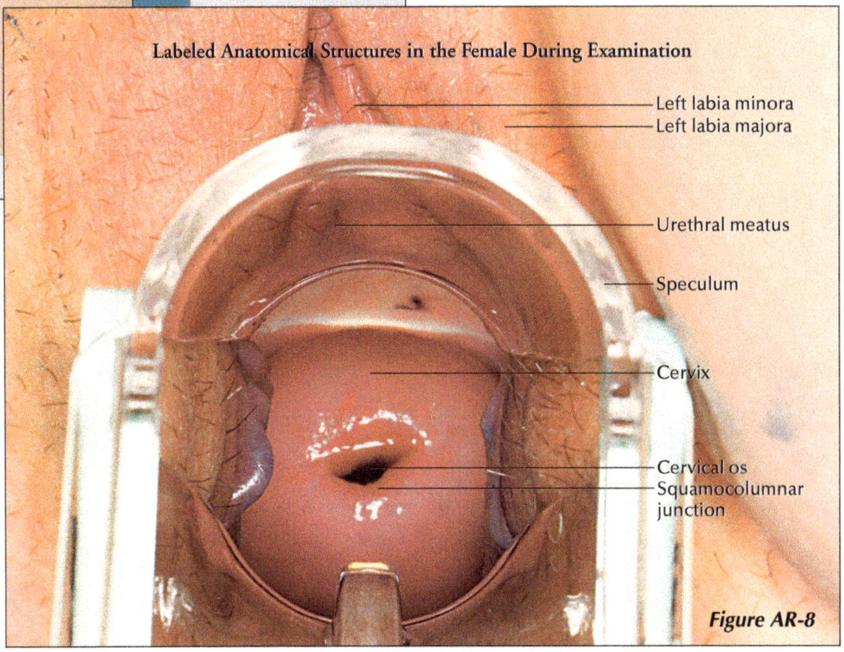

Figure AR-8

DEFINITIONS *(continued)*

— ***Speculum:*** An instrument for opening or distending an orifice to permit visual inspection.

— ***Squamocolumnar junction:*** A clinically visible line demarcating nonkeratinized squamous epithellia from simple columnar cells in the cervical canal.

— ***Urethral meatus:*** A location on the urethra that encircles the lumen of the external opening of the urethral tube. The urethra connects the urinary bladder to the urethral meatus for the purpose of releasing urine.

— ***Vagina:*** The muscular canal, usually 6 to 7 inches in length, extending from the cervix to the hymen. Its walls are lined with squamous cells, creating a mucous membrane with a pH range of 3.8 to 4.5.

— ***Vaginal fornix:*** The protrusion of the cervix into the upper vagina creates vault-like recesses known as the anterior fornix and posterior fornix.

— ***Vaginal introitus:*** Opening of the vagina.

— ***Vaginal vault:*** The enlargement of the internal end of the vagina.

— ***Vaginal vestibule:*** An anatomical area containing the openings of the vagina, urethra, and Bartholin's glands. Anatomical boundaries include the clitoris anteriorly, the labia laterally, and the posterior fourchette posteriorly.

Ano-Rectal

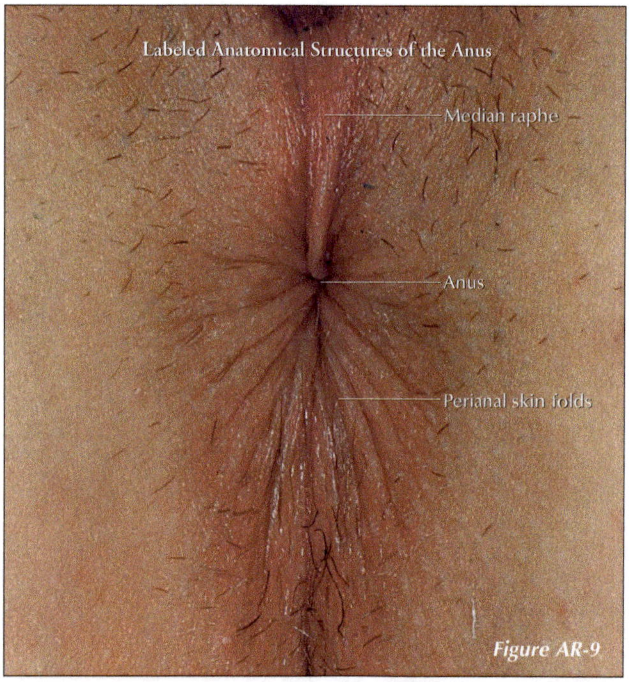

Figure AR-9

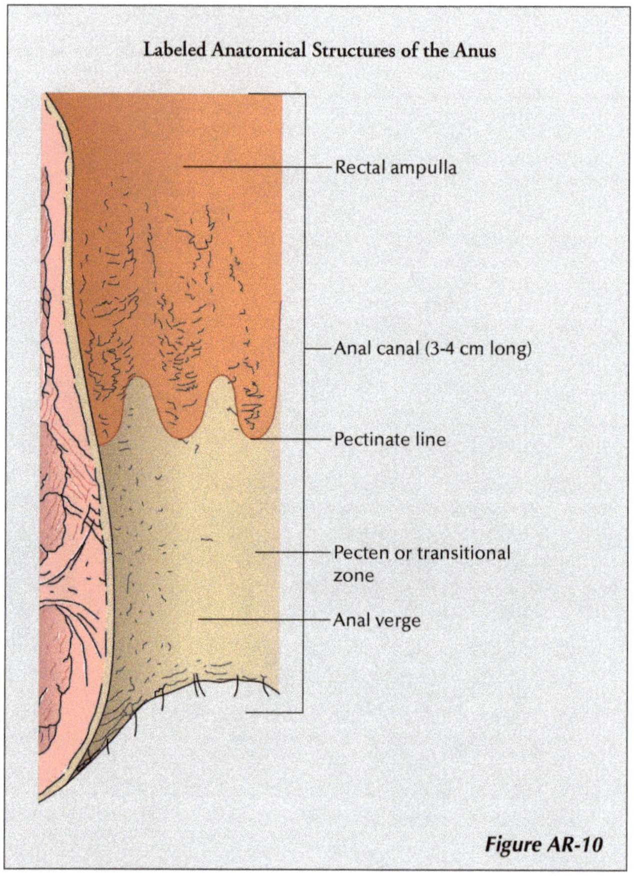

Figure AR-10

Definitions

— ***Anal canal:*** Terminal part of the large intestine, 3 to 4 cm. in length, sensitive to pain, surrounded by sphincter muscles, and without lubricating glands.

— ***Anal verge:*** The distal end of the anal canal, overlies the subcutaneous tissue of the external anal sphincter and extends exteriorly to the margin of anal skin.

— ***Anus:*** The opening of the anal canal, lying between the buttocks, viewed as a linear, slit-like opening, visible with retraction of the buttocks.

— ***Median raphe:*** A visible line of tissue extending from the anus to the perineum. The median raphe is located between the vestibule and the anus in the female and the scrotum and the anus in the male.

— ***Pectinate line*** (also known as dentate line): The saw-toothed line of demarcation between the lower portion of the anal verge and the pectin, a smooth zone of stratified squamous epithelium extending to the anal verge.

— ***Perianal skin folds:*** Wrinkles of perianal skin created by the contraction of the anal sphincter.

— ***Perianal venous engorgement:*** The pooling of venous blood in the circumferential veins of the anus, marked by a bulging of the veins and flat, purple discoloration of the perianal tissues.

— ***Rectal ampulla:*** The proximal portion of the rectum that dilates when the anus opens.

— ***Rectum:*** The distal portion of the large intestine, beginning anterior to the third sacral vertebra.

Chapter 1

Sexual Assault: 41-year-old Female Patient with Down's Syndrome

Objectives

After completing the exercises presented in this chapter, the student will be able to:

1. *Correctly identify the anogenital anatomy of a 41-year-old female patient.*
2. *Identify and document injuries based on an analysis of case photographs.*
3. *List at least 3 items of evidence that should be collected.*
4. *Discuss treatment options based on the patient's history.*

Case History

Mary is a 41-year-old woman with Down's syndrome. Her sister and a law enforcement officer accompany her to the hospital-based SART for a medical forensic examination. Mary is morbidly obese, has the cognitive skills of a child 11 to 12 years of age, and lives with her aunt at her aunt's home. Mary's sister, Lisa, is her legal guardian. Lisa sits next to Mary during the medical forensic interview and examination. During the history, Mary tells the forensic nurse that Bob, a family friend, came to visit her at her aunt's home. She said she was in her bedroom when Bob came in, tied her up, and got on top of her. She says, "He put his t-t in my mouth and v place" and points to the area between her legs when saying "v place." Mary becomes agitated and repeatedly mumbles, "He tied me up." Her motions become increasingly demonstrative and include standing, putting her hands on her waist, and thrusting her hips forward repeatedly, while saying "this is what Bob did." Lisa tries to calm Mary but is unsuccessful. Lisa believes Mary thinks she's in trouble. The forensic nurse reassures Mary she is not in any trouble, and Mary begins to calm and returns to her chair. Each part of the medical forensic examination is explained to Mary, and the nurse answers her questions. Mary is curious about how the nurse will swab her "v place" and what the Toluidine Blue Dye looks like. The nurse shows Mary the cotton-tipped applicators and blue liquid and explains further. Mary says "yes," and her sister signs the consent paperwork. The nurse proceeds with the medical forensic examination and continues to communicate with Mary in a manner she can understand.

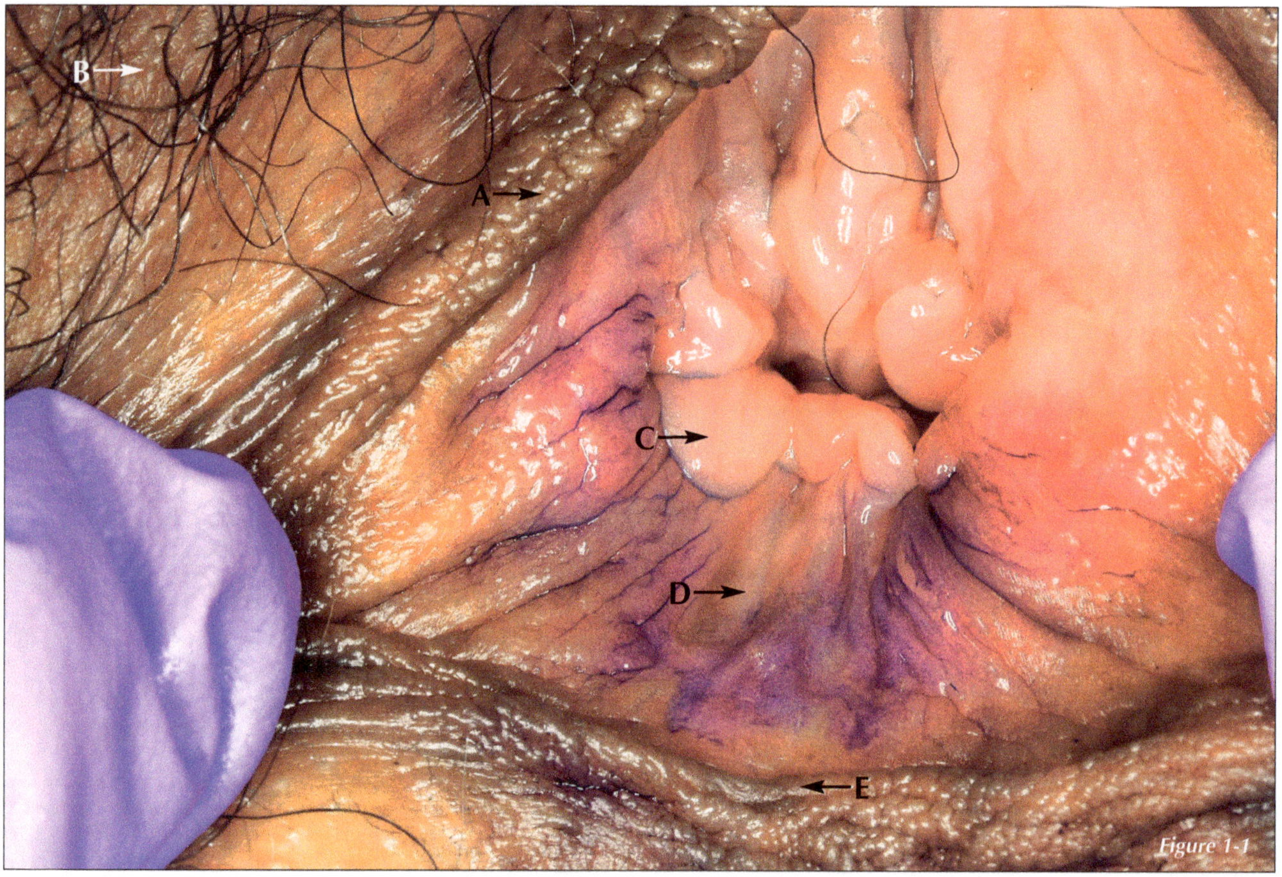

Anatomical Skills 1-1

Refer to **Figure 1-1**. Name the corresponding anatomical locations.

Arrow A: ______________________________

Arrow B: ______________________________

Arrow C: ______________________________

Arrow D: ______________________________

Arrow E: ______________________________

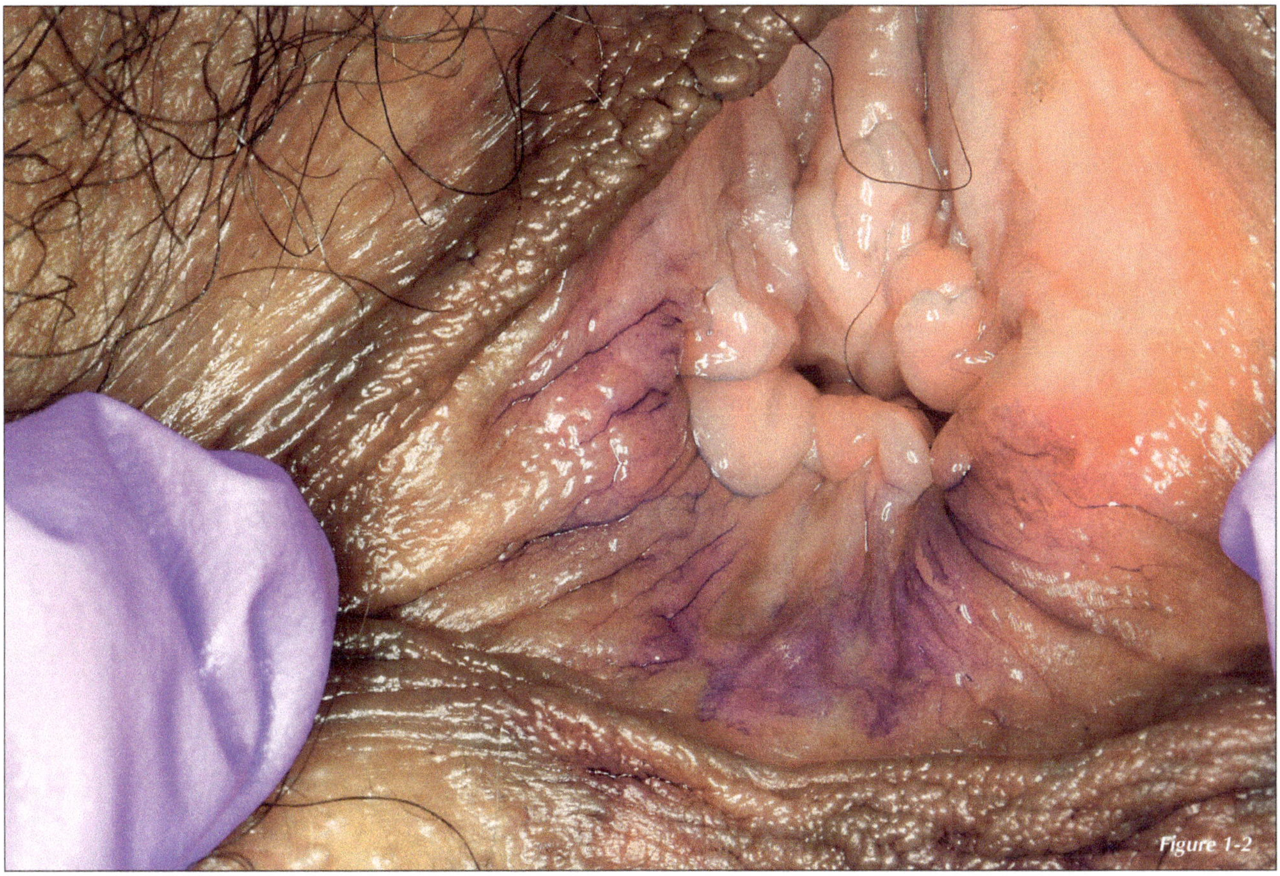

Figure 1-2

Activities 1-1, 1-2, and 1-3

Activity 1-1. Injury Identification

Refer to **Figure 1-2**. Identify any injuries in respect to their anatomical location. Give objective descriptions when documenting findings.

Activity 1-2. Evidence Collection

Using the history and photographs provided, list the evidence you will collect from the patient. Please list the evidence in the order it will be collected.

Activity 1-3. Treatment

Describe the treatment you will offer the patient based on her history and your findings.

Chapter 2

Sexual Assault: 32-year-old Male Patient

Objectives

After completing the exercises presented in this chapter, the student will be able to:

1. *Correctly identify the anogenital anatomy of a 32-year-old male patient.*
2. *Identify and document injuries based on an analysis of case photographs.*
3. *List at least 3 items of evidence that should be collected.*
4. *Discuss treatment options based on the patient's history.*

Case History

Jason is a 32-year-old man who works in the entertainment industry. He shuffles into the emergency department and is taken to the triage desk. He tells the triage nurse, "I have a washcloth up my ass" and explains it is to stop the bleeding. When the triage nurse asks what happened, Jason says, "I was assaulted by this guy I met over the Internet." For several months, he and this man had been having conversations over the Internet. They decided to get together in person for the first time this night. Jason says they were drinking rum and cokes at the bar and the man was getting "rather drunk." After a while, they decided to go out to the man's car. While in the backseat of the car, the two men engaged in consensual heavy petting, including performing and receiving fellatio. When Jason refused to let the man anally penetrate him with his fingers, the man became aggressive and "fisted" him. Jason drove to the emergency department unaccompanied to seek care.

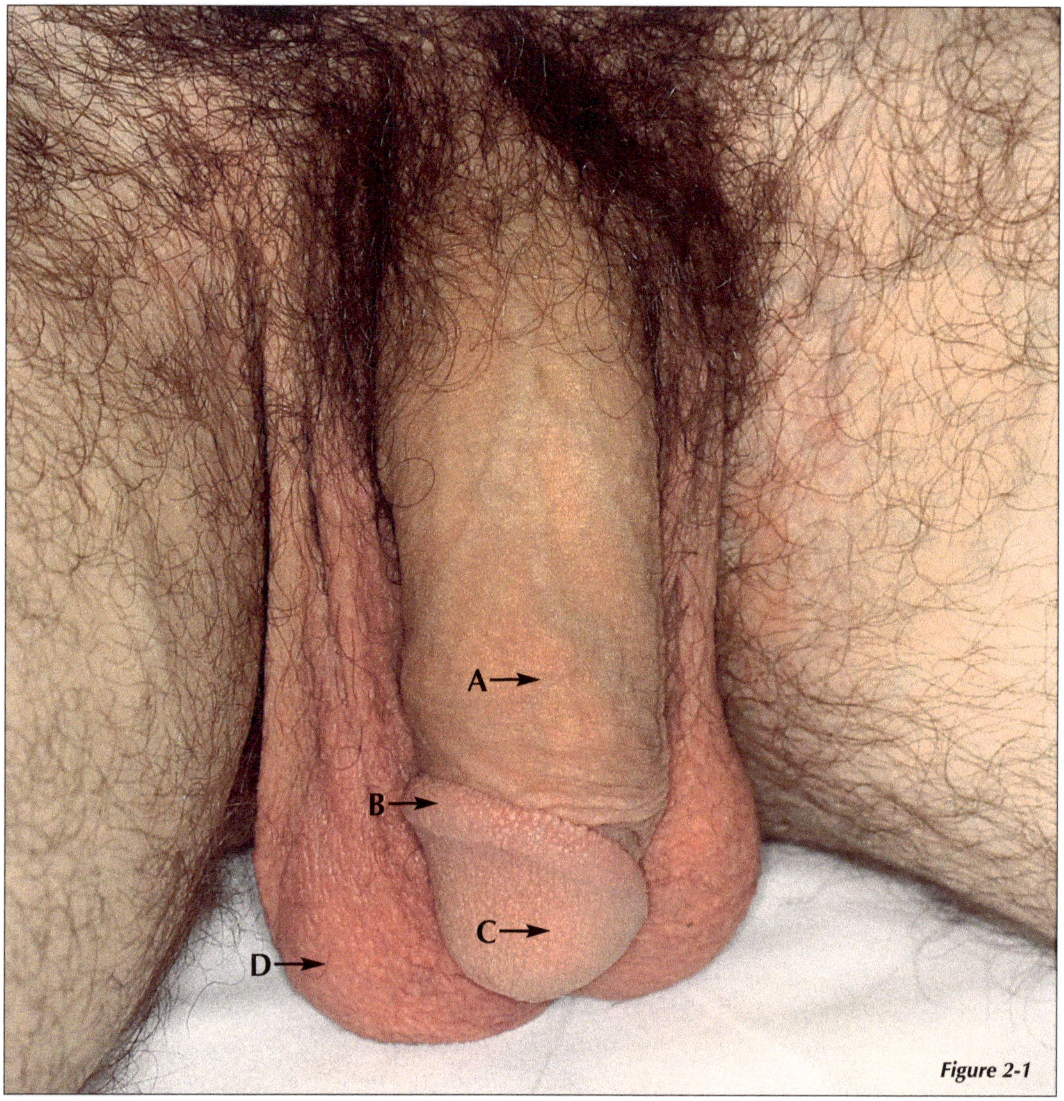

Figure 2-1

Anatomical Skills 2-1

Refer to **Figure 2-1**. Name the corresponding anatomical locations.

Arrow A: ______________________________

Arrow B: ______________________________

Arrow C: ______________________________

Arrow D: ______________________________

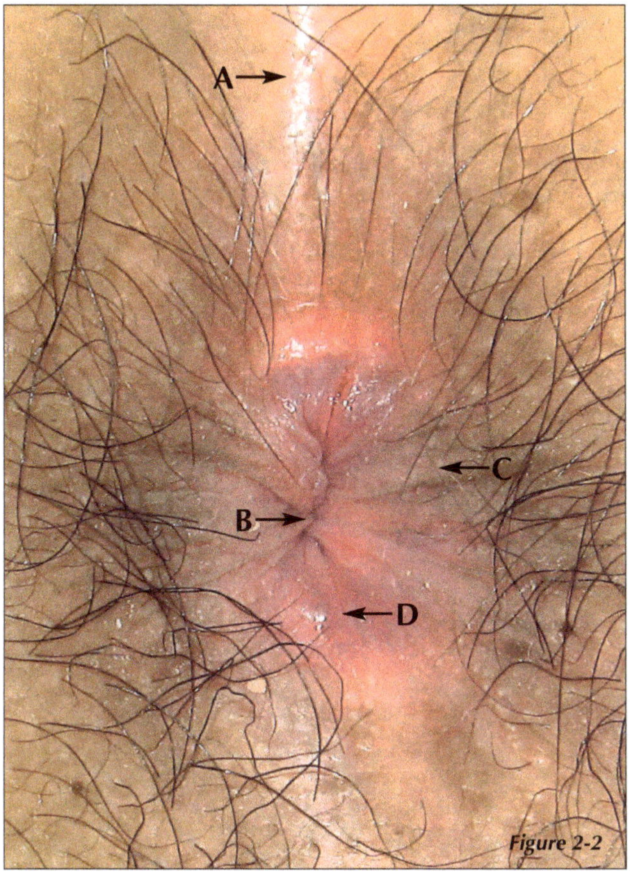

Anatomical Skills 2-2

Refer to **Figure 2-2**. Name the corresponding anatomical locations.

Arrow A: ______________________________

Arrow B: ______________________________

Arrow C: ______________________________

Arrow D: ______________________________

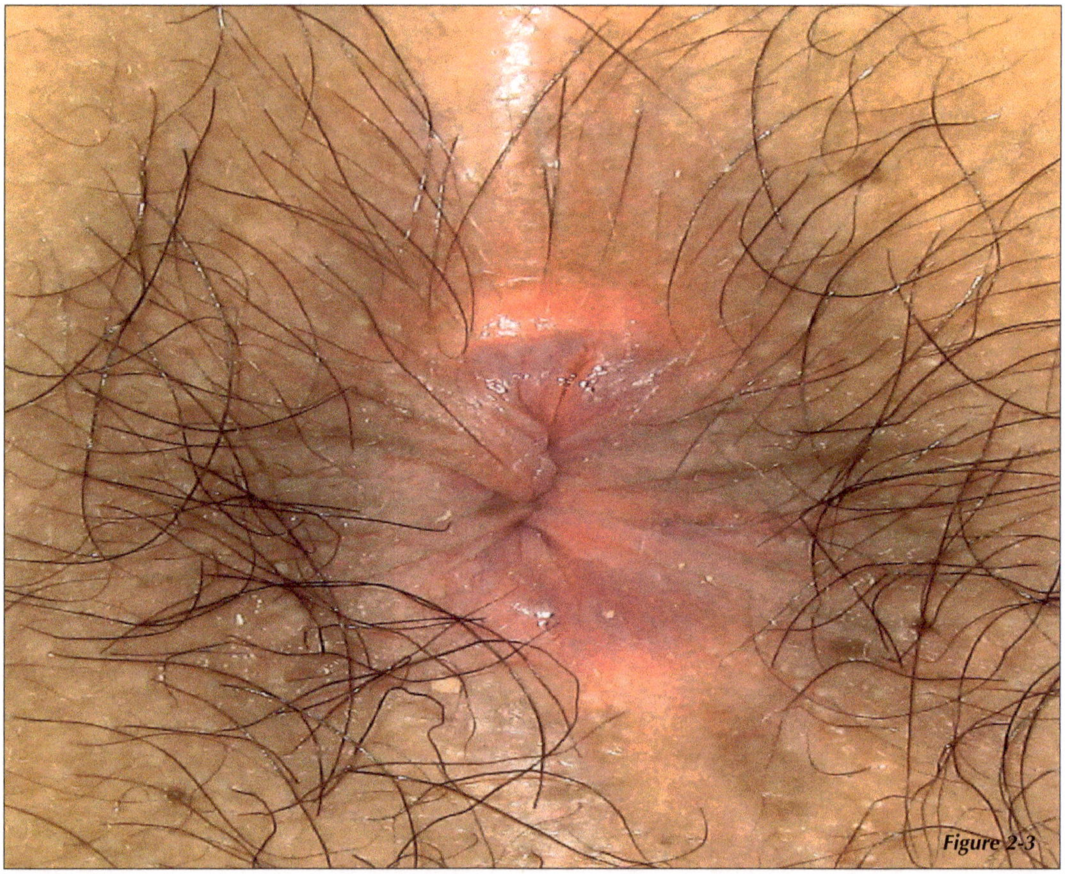

Figure 2-3

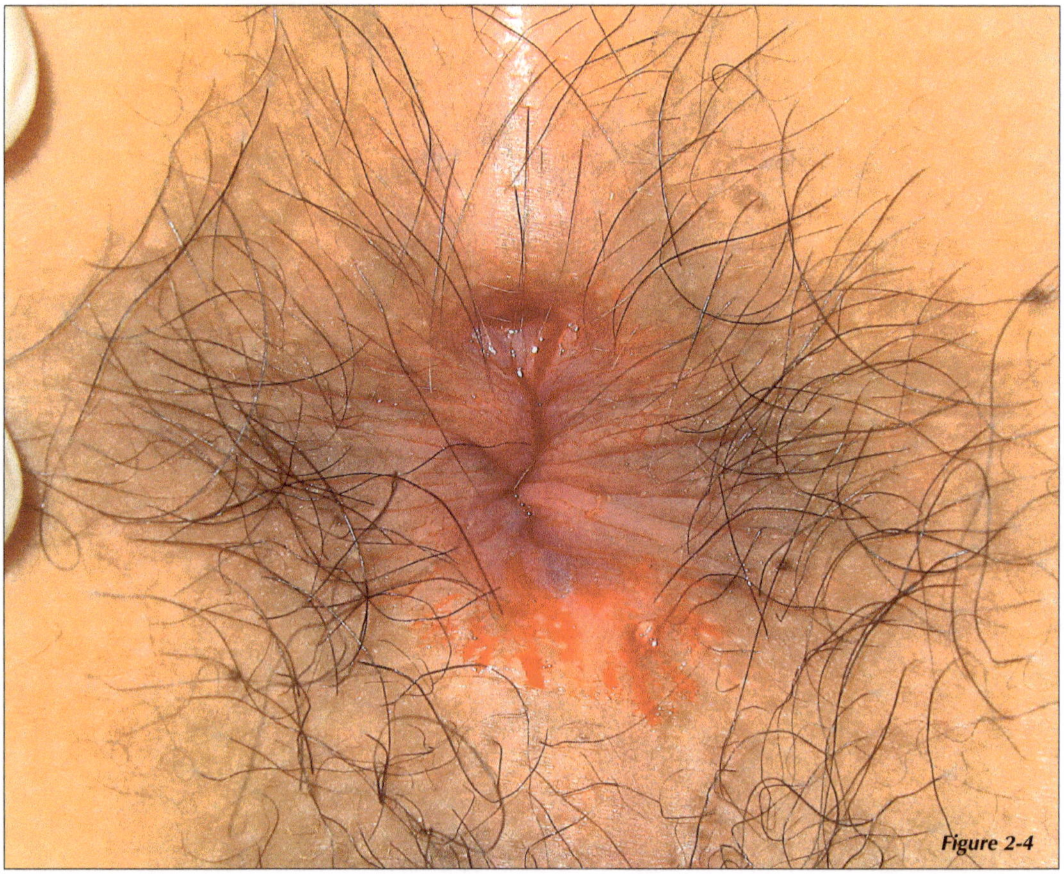

Figure 2-4

Activities 2-1, 2-2, and 2-3

Activity 2-1. Injury Identification

Refer to **Figures 2-3** and **2-4**. Identify any injuries in respect to their anatomical location. Give objective descriptions when documenting findings.

Activity 2-2. Evidence Collection

Using the history and photographs provided, list the evidence you will collect from the patient. Please list the evidence in the order it will be collected.

Activity 2-3. Treatment

Describe the treatment you will offer the patient based on his history and your findings.

Chapter 3

Incapacitated Sexual Assault: 24-year-old Female Patient

Objectives

After completing the exercises presented in this chapter, the student will be able to:

1. *Correctly identify the anogenital anatomy of a 24-year-old female patient.*
2. *Identify and document injuries based on an analysis of case photographs.*
3. *List at least 3 items of evidence that should be collected.*
4. *Discuss treatment options based on the patient's history.*

Case History

Rebecca is a 24-year-old woman who works as an interior designer for a large company. She has never been pregnant, and her last sexual activity was almost two months ago. When asked about alcohol intake, Rebecca says, "I like to party just like any other girl my age. I drink a lot, but only when I go out with my friends." Rebecca says she was with her coworkers last night and remembers accepting a drink from her boss. She cannot recall anything that happened between the time she accepted the drink and waking up early this morning sitting up on her boss's couch. Her boss told her she got drunk at the party and he took her to his apartment where she "would be safe to sleep it off." Rebecca told her boss, "I feel like something happened down there," and he assured her nothing happened. She then accepted his offer to take her home. Rebecca says, "My mother was frantic when I got home because I never stay out all night. I told her I thought something happened, and she said I should come here to see if he raped me."

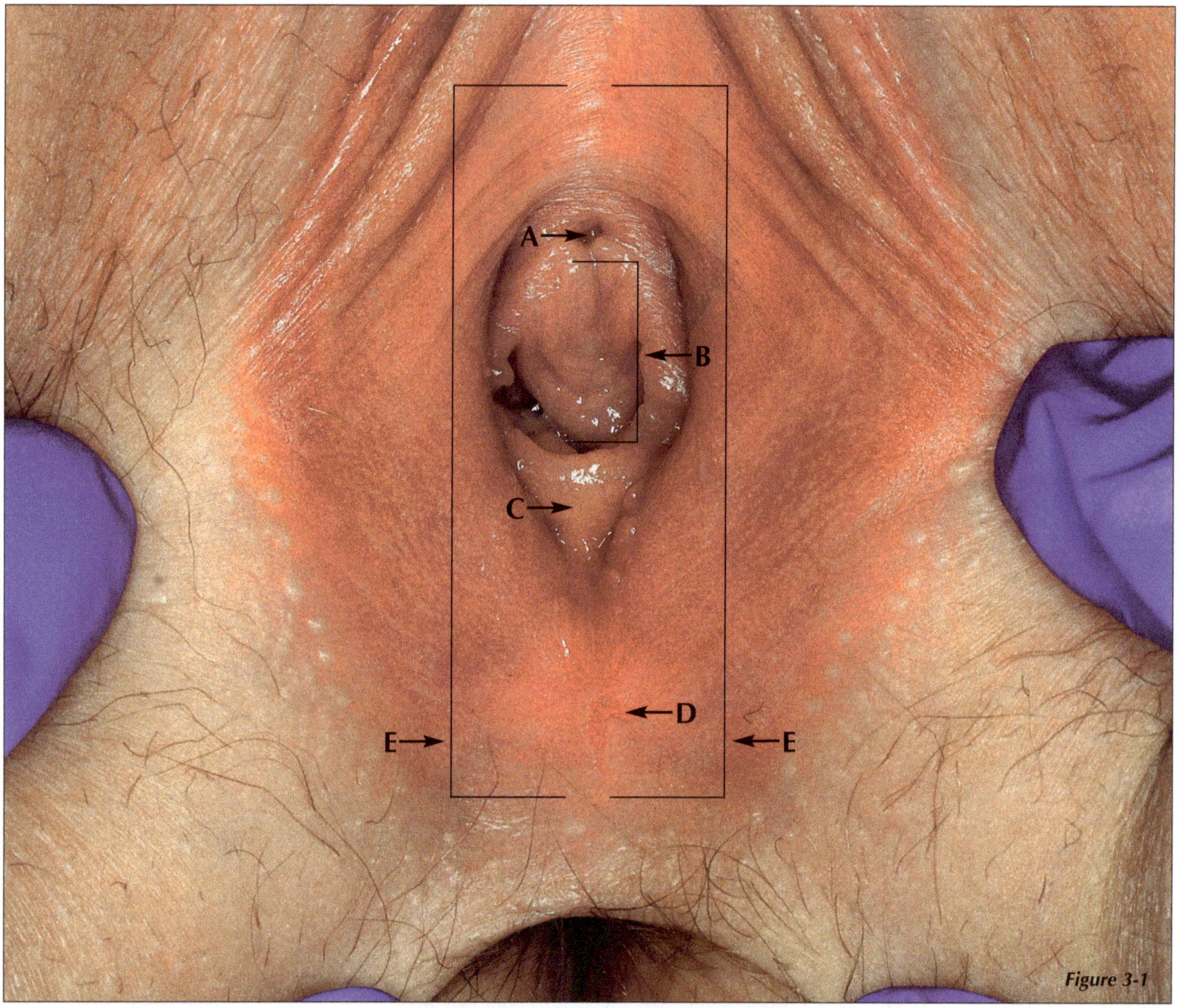

Anatomical Skills 3-1

Refer to **Figure 3-1**. Name the corresponding anatomical locations.

Arrow A: ______________________________

Arrow B: ______________________________

Arrow C: ______________________________

Arrow D: ______________________________

Arrow E: ______________________________

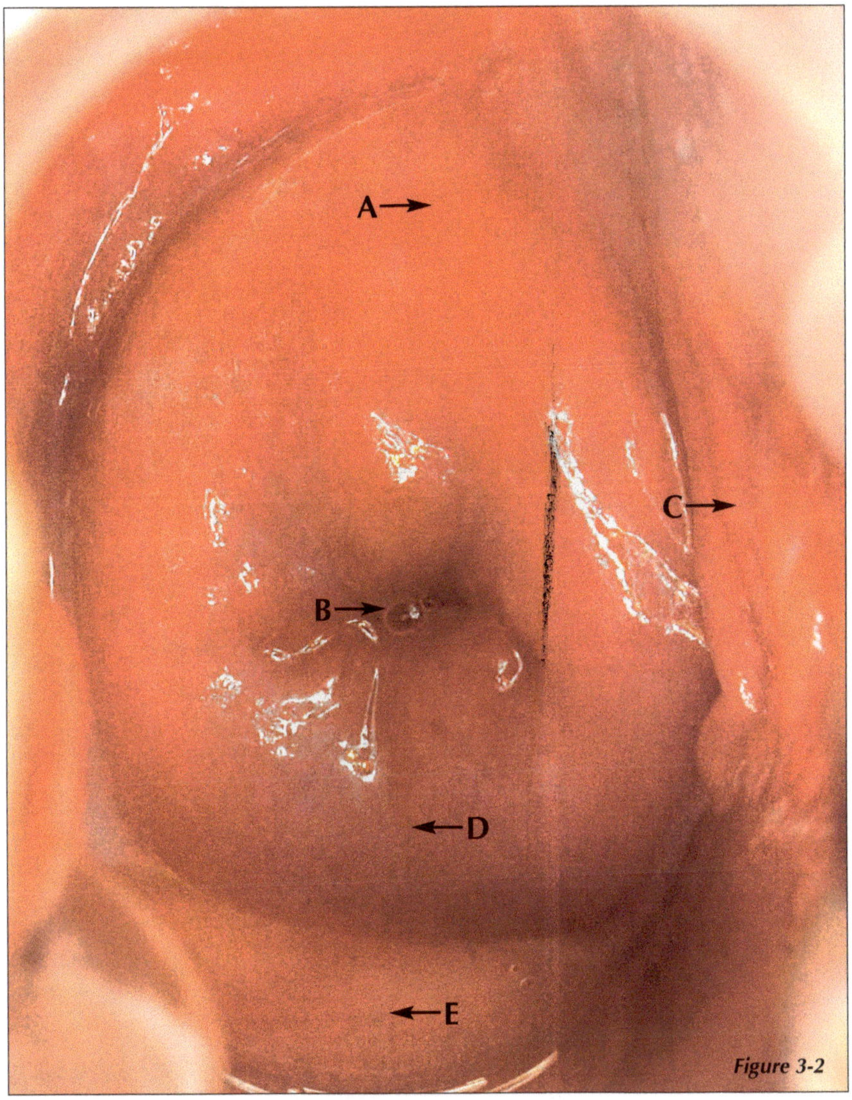

Figure 3-2

Anatomical Skills 3-2

Refer to **Figure 3-2**. Name the corresponding anatomical locations.

Arrow A: ______________________________

Arrow B: ______________________________

Arrow C: ______________________________

Arrow D: ______________________________

Arrow E: ______________________________

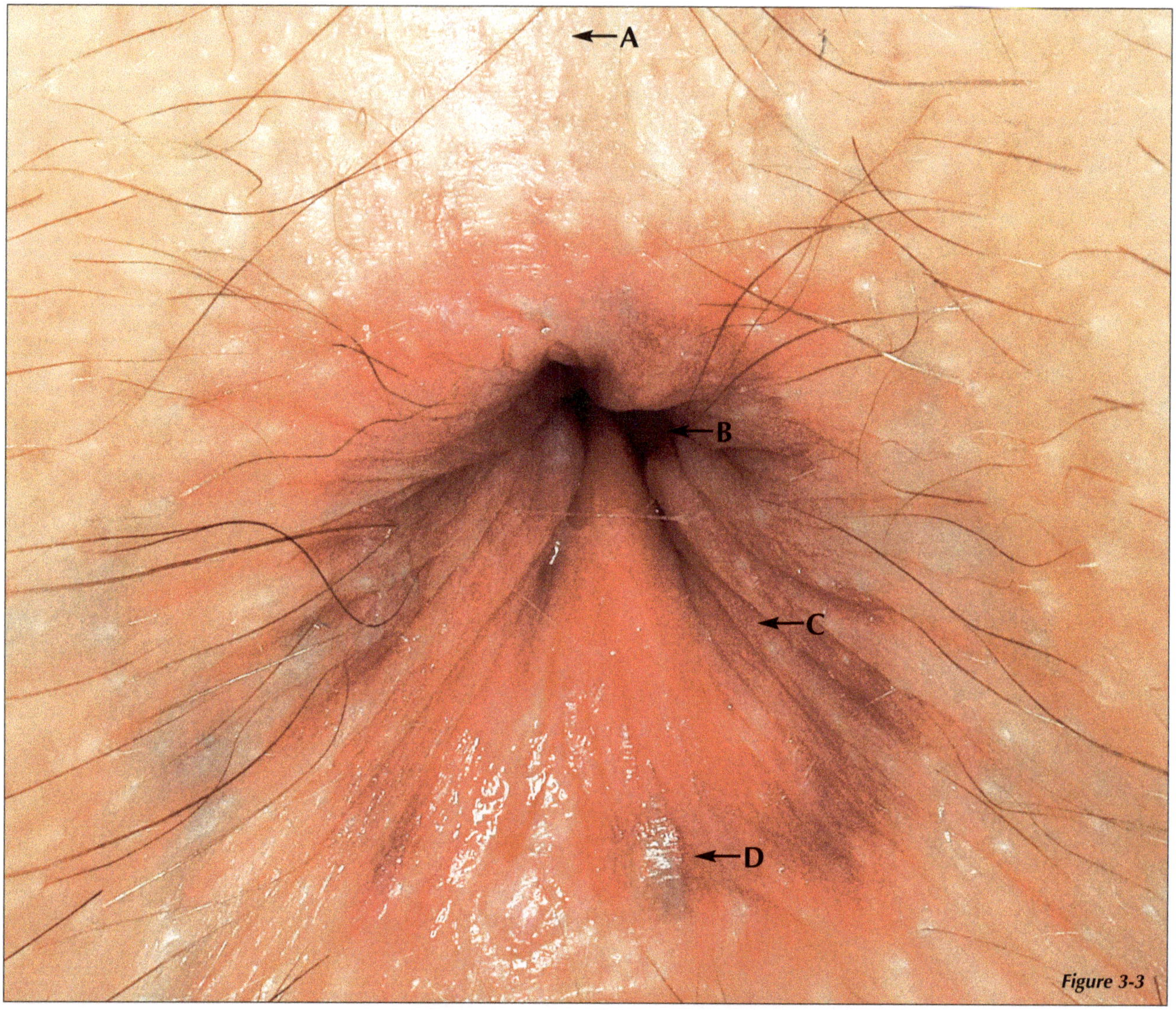

Figure 3-3

Anatomical Skills 3-3

Refer to **Figure 3-3**. Name the corresponding anatomical locations.

Arrow A: ______________________________

Arrow B: ______________________________

Arrow C: ______________________________

Arrow D: ______________________________

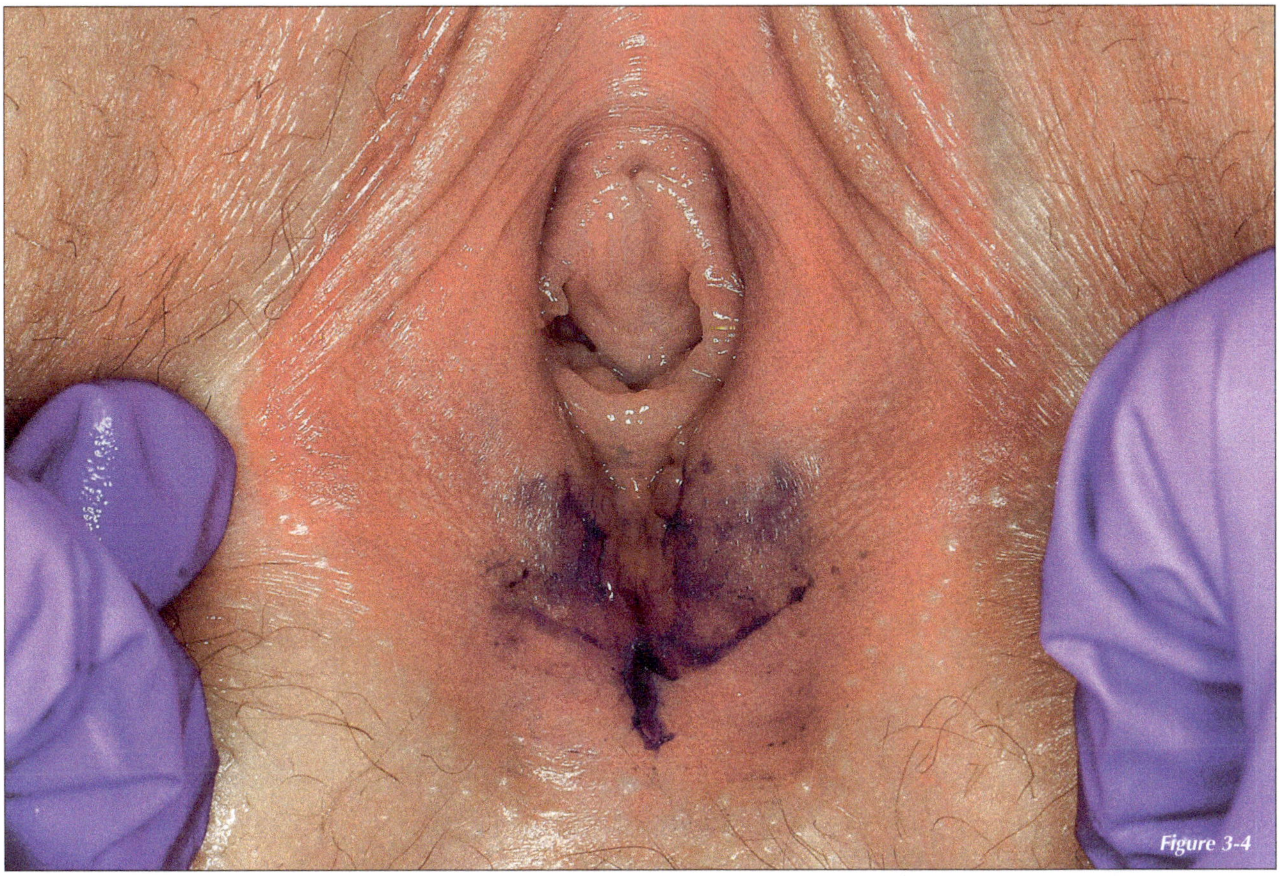

Figure 3-4

Activities 3-1, 3-2, 3-3, 3-4, and 3-5

Activity 3-1. Injury Identification

Refer to **Figure 3-4**. Identify any injuries in respect to their anatomical location. Give objective descriptions when documenting findings.

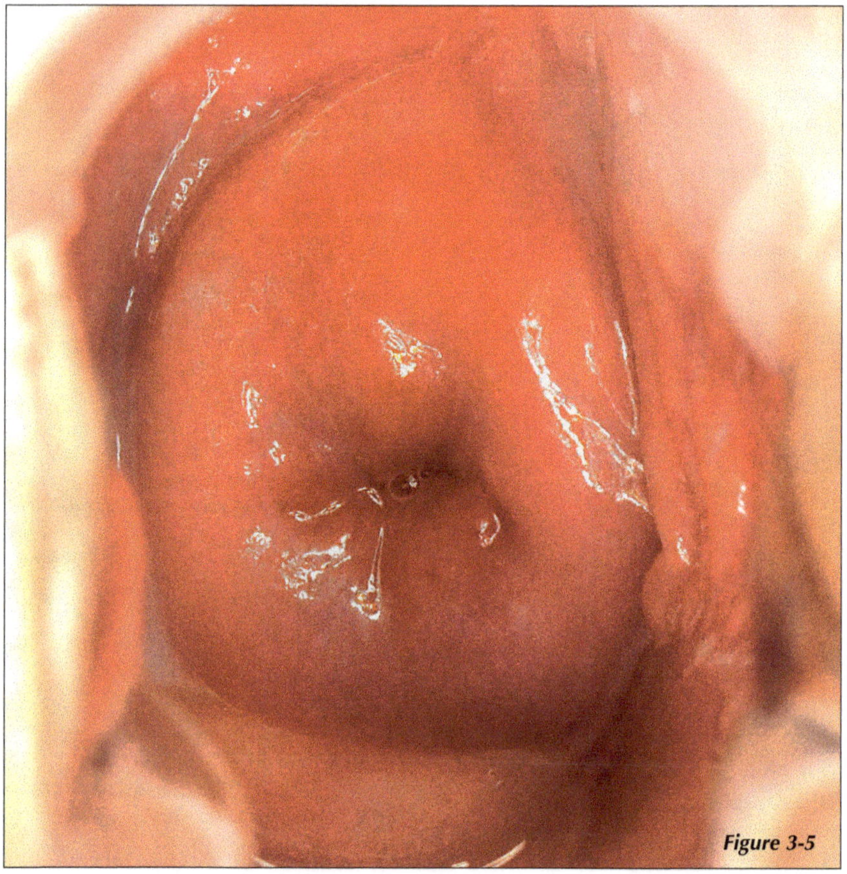

Figure 3-5

ACTIVITY 3-2. INJURY IDENTIFICATION

Refer to **Figure 3-5**. Identify any injuries in respect to their anatomical location. Give objective descriptions when documenting findings.

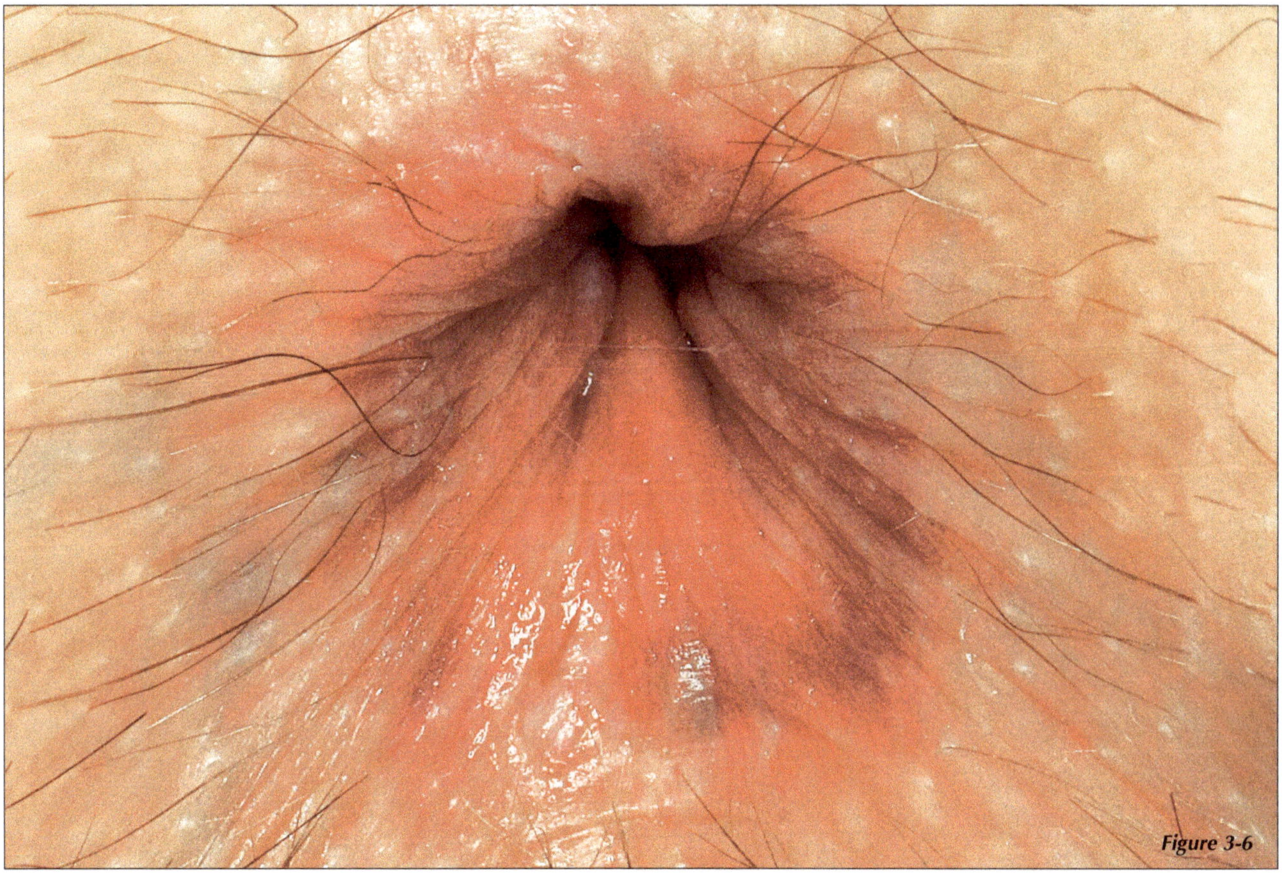

Figure 3-6

ACTIVITY 3-3. INJURY IDENTIFICATION

Refer to **Figure 3-6**. Identify any injuries in respect to their anatomical location. Give objective descriptions when documenting findings.

Activity 3-4. Evidence Collection

Using the history and photographs provided, list the evidence you will collect from the patient. Please list the evidence in the order it will be collected.

Activity 3-5. Treatment

Describe the treatment you will offer the patient based on her history and your findings.

Chapter 4

SEXUAL ASSAULT: 21-YEAR-OLD FEMALE COLLEGE STUDENT

OBJECTIVES

After completing the exercises presented in this chapter, the student will be able to:

1. *Correctly identify the anogenital and oral anatomy of a 21-year-old female patient.*
2. *Identify and document injuries based on an analysis of case photographs.*
3. *List at least 3 items of evidence that should be collected.*
4. *Discuss treatment options based on the patient's history.*

CASE HISTORY

Jenny is a 21-year-old college student who lives off campus. Her apartment air conditioner does not work, and the temperatures have been hovering around 100 degrees during the day. To stay cool at night, Jenny has been opening her window, turning on the fan, and falling asleep. This morning around 3:00AM she woke up and saw a man crawling on the floor of her bedroom. When the man saw she had awakened, he stood and put a gun to her head and told her not to scream. He told her to turn over onto her stomach and proceeded to penetrate her vaginally with his penis. After multiple thrusts he withdrew his penis, rolled her over onto her back, and yelled, "Open your mouth bitch." Jenny tells the forensic nurse she was scared and then says, "I did what he told me to do, and I opened my mouth. Then he shoved it [penis] in my mouth and told me to do it right. When he came, he put the gun to my head and said, 'Swallow it bitch.'" The man then told her not to move, and he quietly left her apartment. Jenny grabbed her phone and ran to the bathroom but was unable to make it to the toilet and vomited on the floor. She then called 911. The police arrived and brought Jenny to the emergency department for a medical forensic evaluation by the forensic nurse.

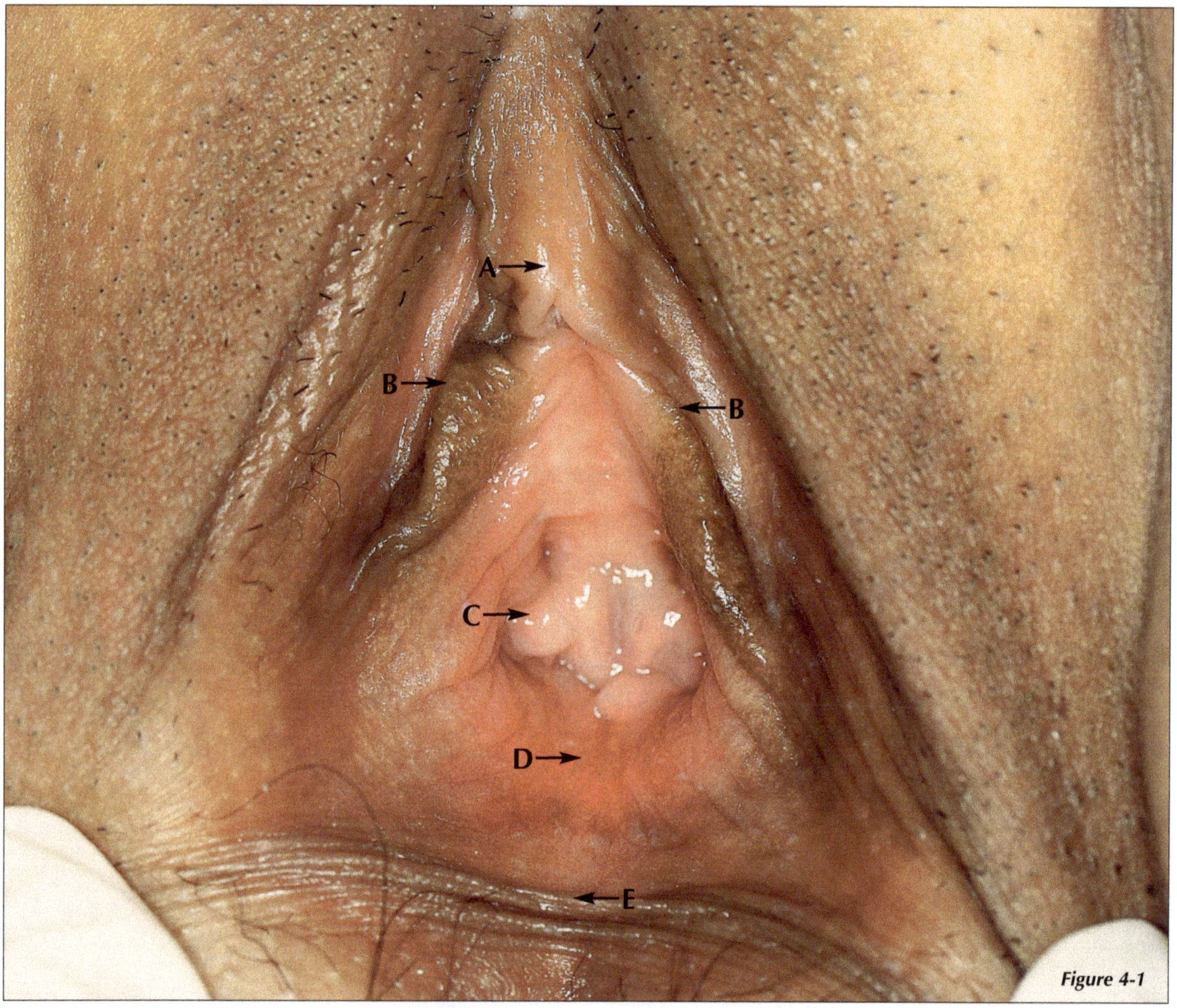

Figure 4-1

Anatomical Skills 4-1

Refer to **Figure 4-1**. Name the corresponding anatomical locations.

Arrow A: ______________________________

Arrow B: ______________________________

Arrow C: ______________________________

Arrow D: ______________________________

Arrow E: ______________________________

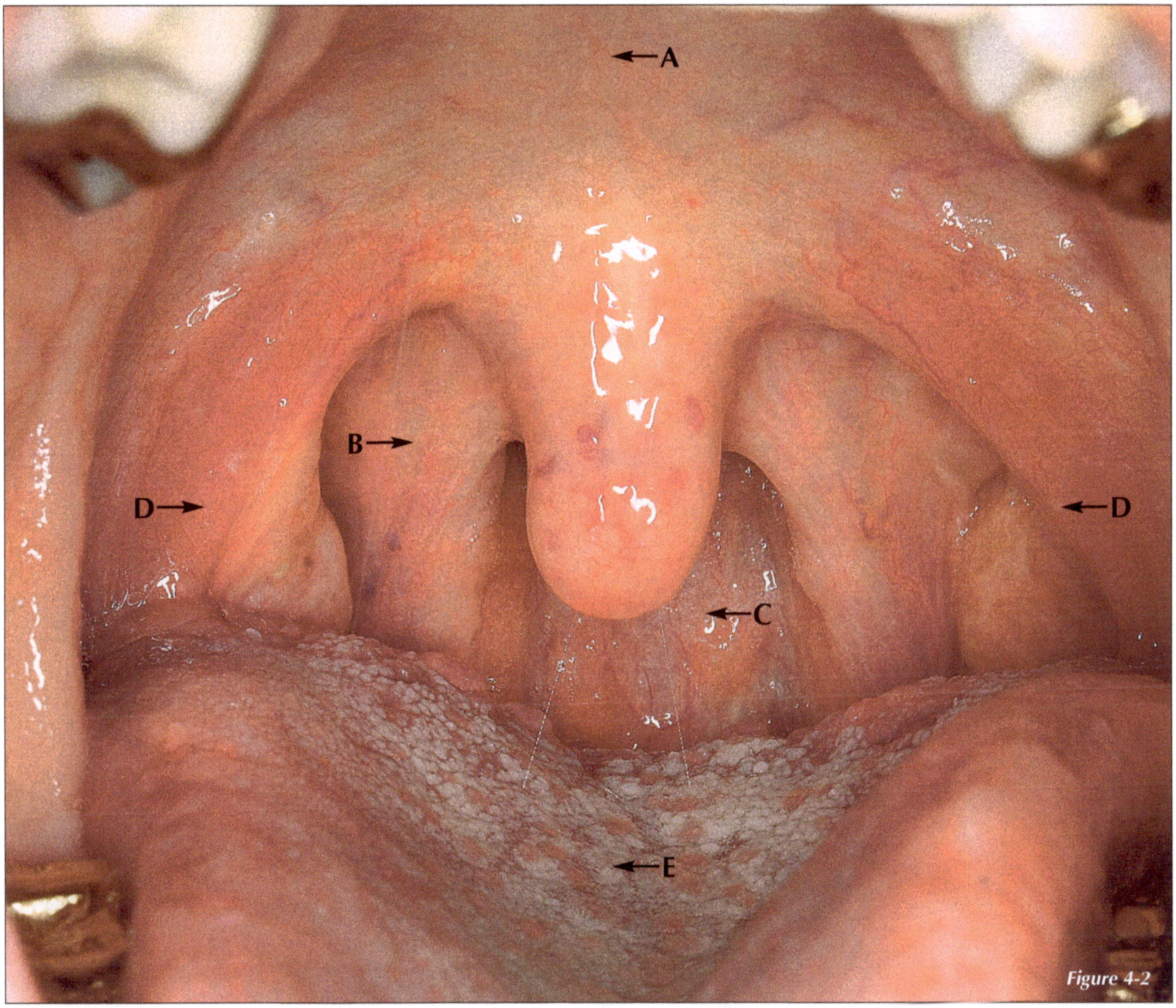

Figure 4-2

Anatomical Skills 4-2

Refer to **Figure 4-2**. Name the corresponding anatomical locations.

Arrow A: ______________________________

Arrow B: ______________________________

Arrow C: ______________________________

Arrow D: ______________________________

Arrow E: ______________________________

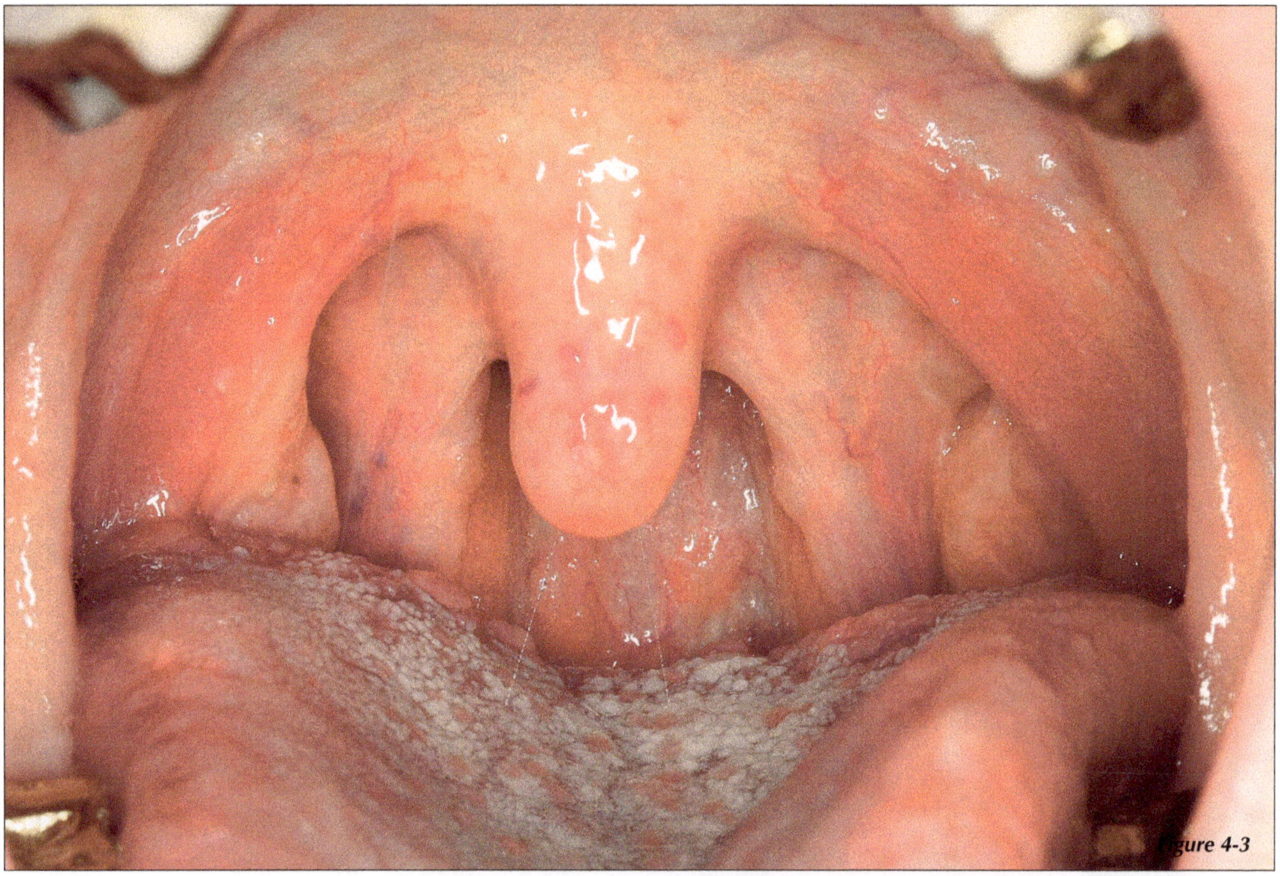

Figure 4-3

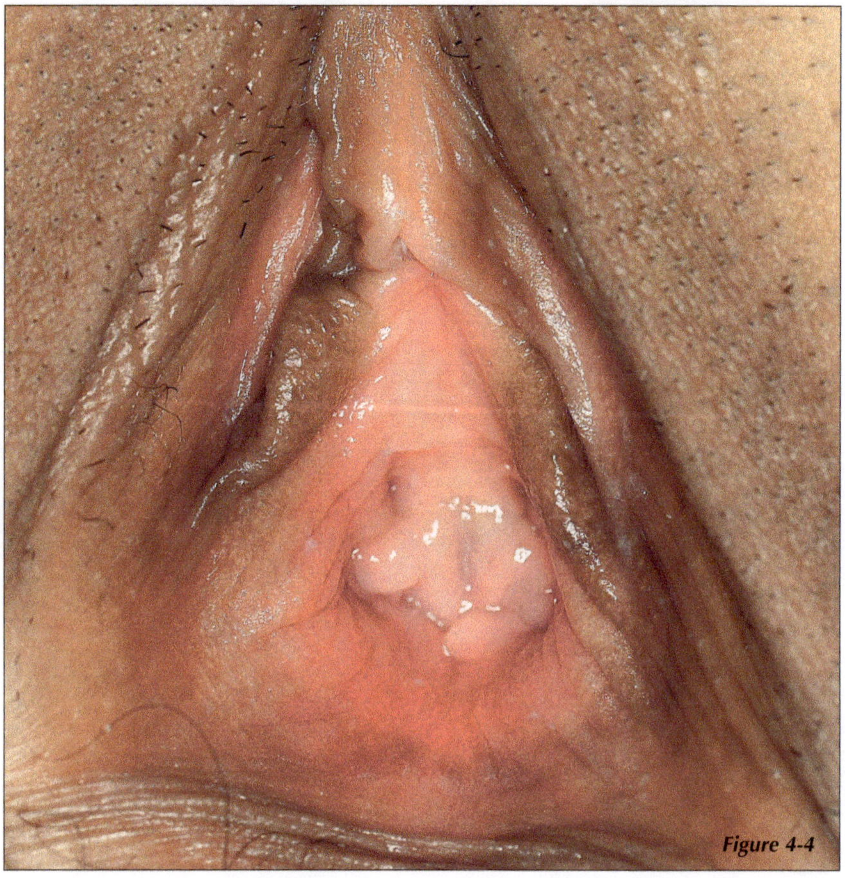

Figure 4-4

Activities 4-1, 4-2, and 4-3

Activity 4-1. Injury Identification

Refer to **Figures 4-3** and **4-4**. Identify any injuries in respect to their anatomical location. Give objective descriptions when documenting findings.

Activity 4-2. Evidence Collection

Using the history and photographs provided, list the evidence you will collect from the patient. Please list the evidence in the order it will be collected.

Activity 4-3. Treatment

Describe the treatment you will offer the patient based on her history and your findings.

Chapter 5

Drug-Facilitated Sexual Assault: 15-year-old Female Patient

Objectives

After completing the exercises presented in this chapter, the student will be able to:

1. *Correctly identify the anogenital anatomy of a 15-year-old female patient.*
2. *Identify and document injuries based on an analysis of case photographs.*
3. *List at least 3 items of evidence that should be collected.*
4. *Discuss treatment options based on the patient's history.*

Case History

Chrystal is a 15-year-old who is doing poorly in school. She was recently re-assigned to home school; however, her studies have been intermittent. Her mother works from late morning to late in the evening, and Chrystal is often home alone. She has several friends who live in her apartment complex. Yesterday Chrystal walked down to Shane's apartment. Shane is 19 years old and Chrystal has known him for about a year. Terrence, a 22-year-old man from the neighborhood, was also there. They started drinking beer followed by several shooters. Chrystal does not usually drink. After one beer and one shooter, she began feeling sick and was having a difficult time focusing. She remembers stumbling into the bedroom to lie down. The next morning, Chrystal's mother realized she was still not home and alerted the neighbors. They immediately started looking for Chrystal, but her mom had to go to work. After learning Chrystal was in Shane's apartment the day before, the neighbors went to his apartment. Terrence was still there. He let them in and told them Chrystal was in the bedroom, but the bedroom door was locked. They forced the door open to find Shane, naked, on top of her. Chrystal was on the bed naked with her legs spread apart; she appeared to be unconscious. She was taken to the hospital and is now awake. Chrystal does not remember anything before waking up this morning in the back of the ambulance. Her mother was called and will be at the hospital within the hour.

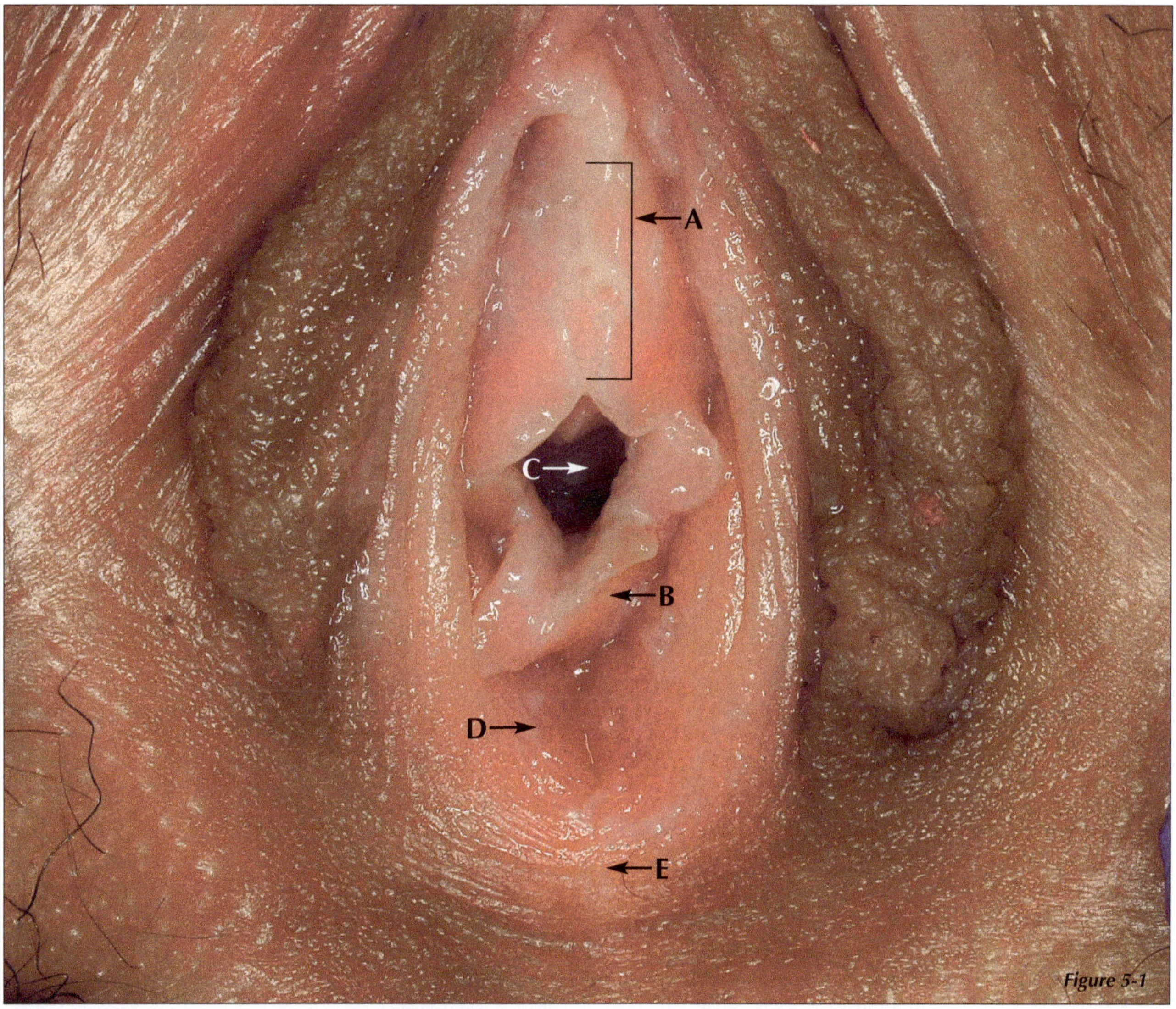

Figure 5-1

ANATOMICAL SKILLS 5-1

Refer to **Figure 5-1**. Name the corresponding anatomical locations.

Arrow A: ______________________________

Arrow B: ______________________________

Arrow C: ______________________________

Arrow D: ______________________________

Arrow E: ______________________________

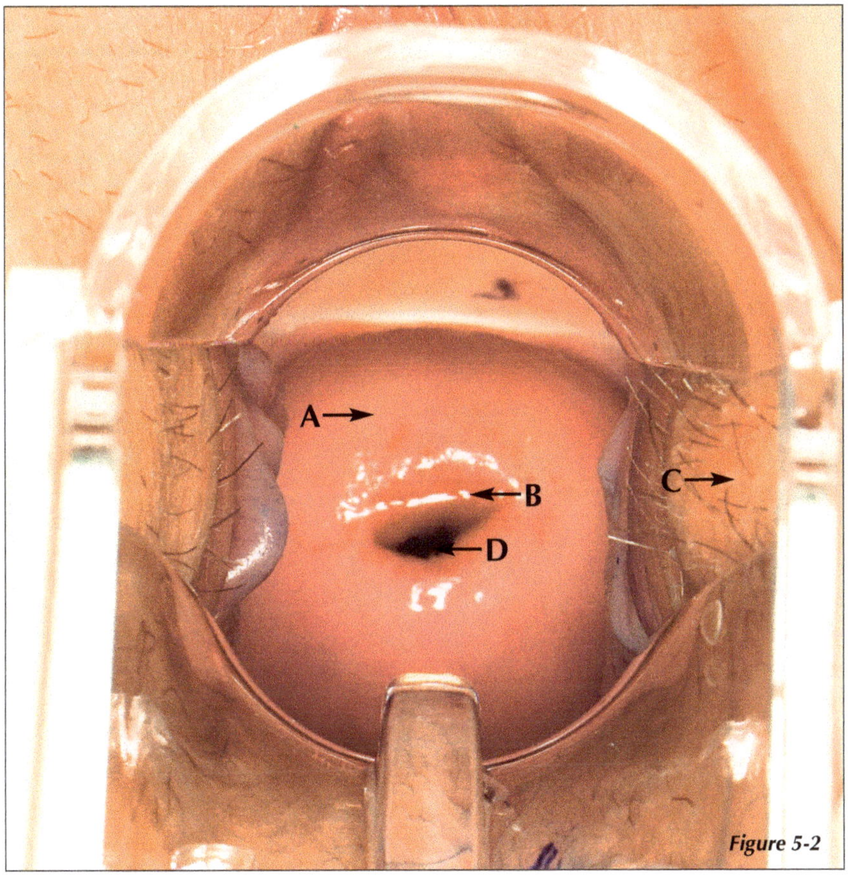

Figure 5-2

Anatomical Skills 5-2

Refer to **Figure 5-2**. Name the corresponding anatomical locations.

Arrow A: ______________________________

Arrow B: ______________________________

Arrow C: ______________________________

Arrow D: ______________________________

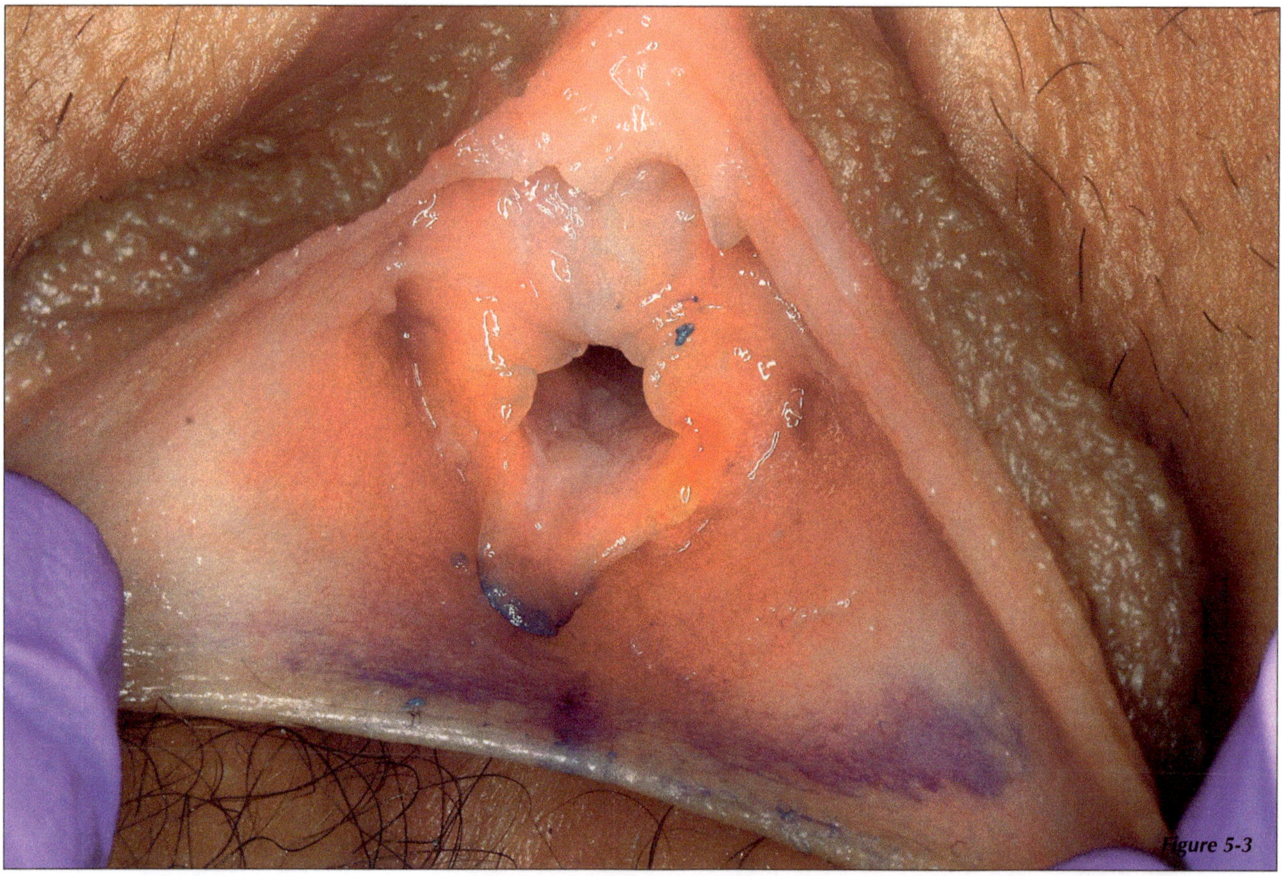

Figure 5-3

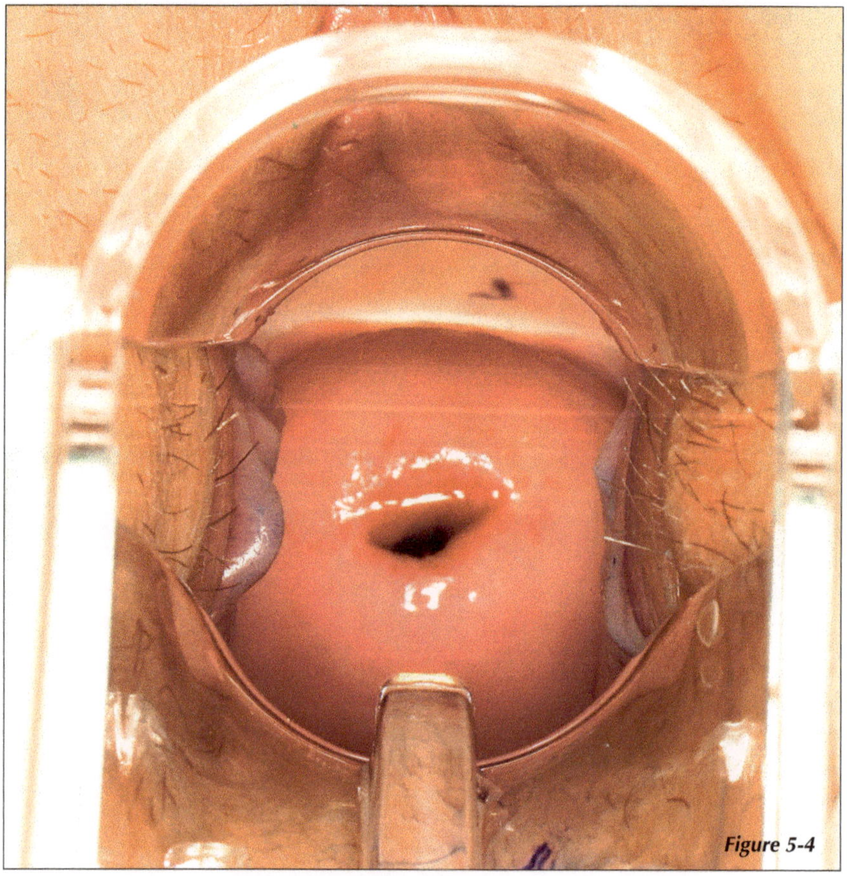

Figure 5-4

Activities 5-1, 5-2, and 5-3

Activity 5-1. Injury Identification

Refer to **Figures 5-3** and **5-4**. Identify any injuries in respect to their anatomical location. Give objective descriptions when documenting findings.

Activity 5-2. Evidence Collection

Using the history and photographs provided, list the evidence you will collect from the patient. Please list the evidence in the order it will be collected.

Activity 5-3. Treatment

Describe the treatment you will offer the patient based on her history and your findings.

Chapter 6

Sexual Assault: 17-year-old Female Patient

Objectives

After completing the exercises presented in this chapter, the student will be able to:

1. *Correctly identify the oral and anogenital anatomy of a 17-year-old female patient.*
2. *Identify and document injuries based on an analysis of case photographs.*
3. *List at least 3 items of evidence that should be collected.*
4. *Discuss treatment options based on the patient's history.*

Case History

Ginna is 17 years old and wants to be a fashion designer. She works after school at an outlet that sells clothing. Earlier this evening, she was completing the clothing inventory before closing when two men entered the store. The men remained at the store until closing and purchased more than $500 of merchandise. They then invited Ginna to go with them to get something to eat. She decided to go and called her family to let them know they would not need to pick her up from work. The two men and Ginna were driving around and talking on their way to Wally's restaurant when the men turned into a driveway and said, "This is where we live. We need to drop the clothes off before we eat." Ginna needed to use the restroom and agreed to accompany them inside. Once inside, they offered her a drink and she declined. One of the men showed her to a restroom down the hallway. While she was in the restroom, the two men pushed the door open, grabbed her, and dragged her to a bedroom. Ginna said she fought until they threw her against the wall and she lost consciousness. When she awoke, her wrists were tied to the bed and "they were raping me." She remembers one of the men saying, "Whore, you better not move." When they were done, they left the room. Ginna broke the ties, crawled out of the house, and ran naked to the next-door neighbor's home. The neighbor immediately called 911. The police arrived, and Ginna was taken by ambulance to the emergency department of a local hospital. The SART was activated.

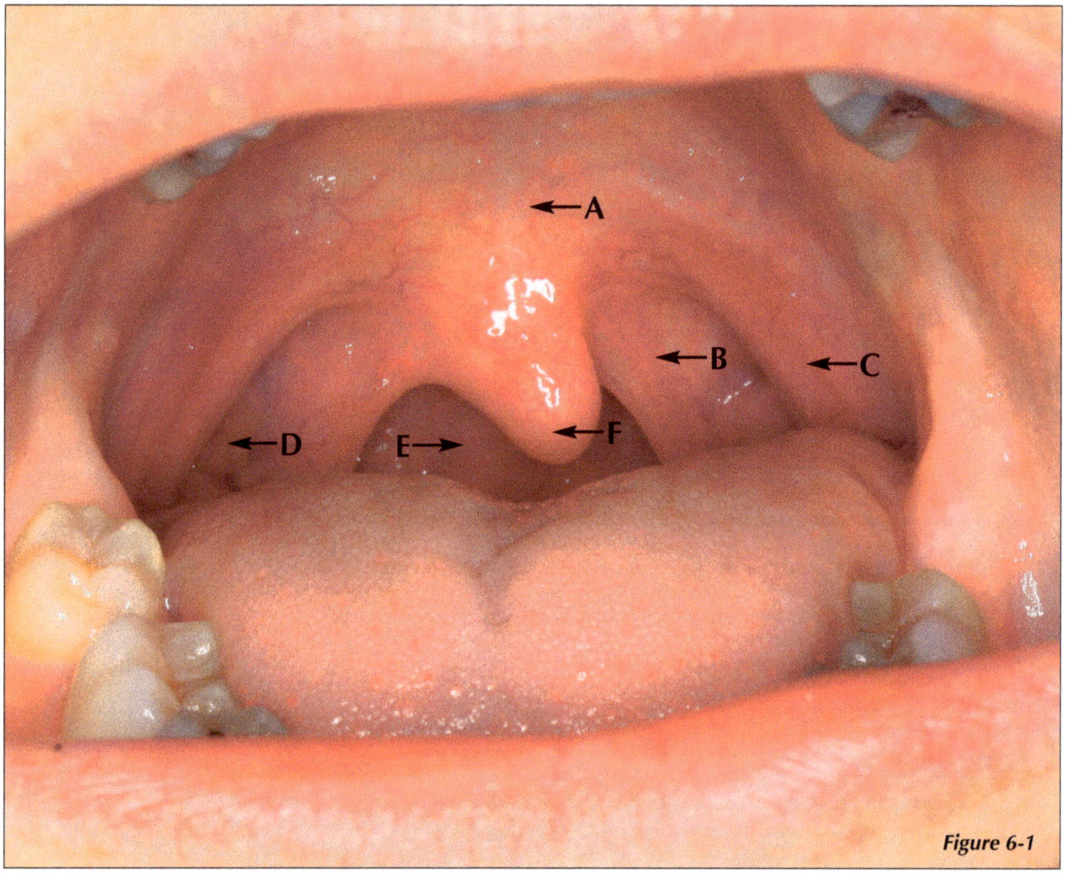

ANATOMICAL SKILLS 6-1

Refer to **Figure 6-1**. Name the corresponding anatomical locations.

Arrow A: ____________________

Arrow B: ____________________

Arrow C: ____________________

Arrow D: ____________________

Arrow E: ____________________

Arrow F: ____________________

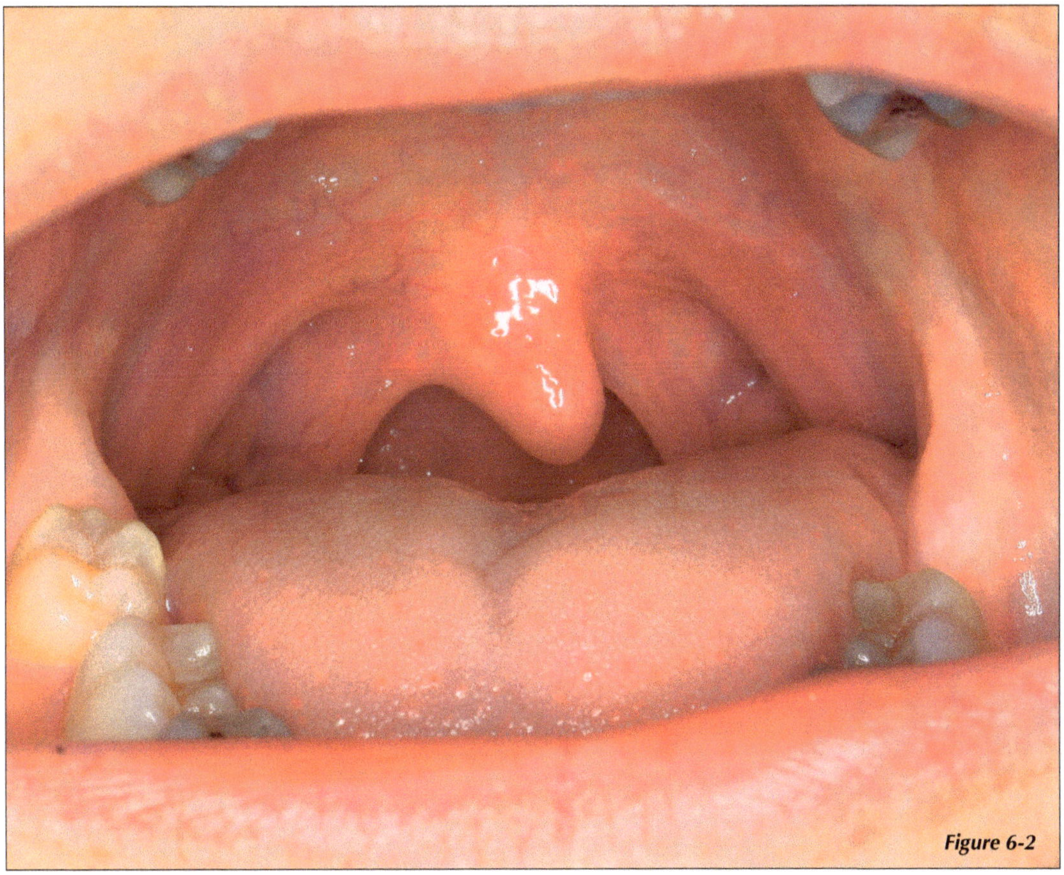

Figure 6-2

Activities 6-1, 6-2, 6-3, and 6-4

Activity 6-1. Injury Identification

Refer to **Figure 6-2**. Identify any injuries in respect to their anatomical location. Give objective descriptions when documenting findings.

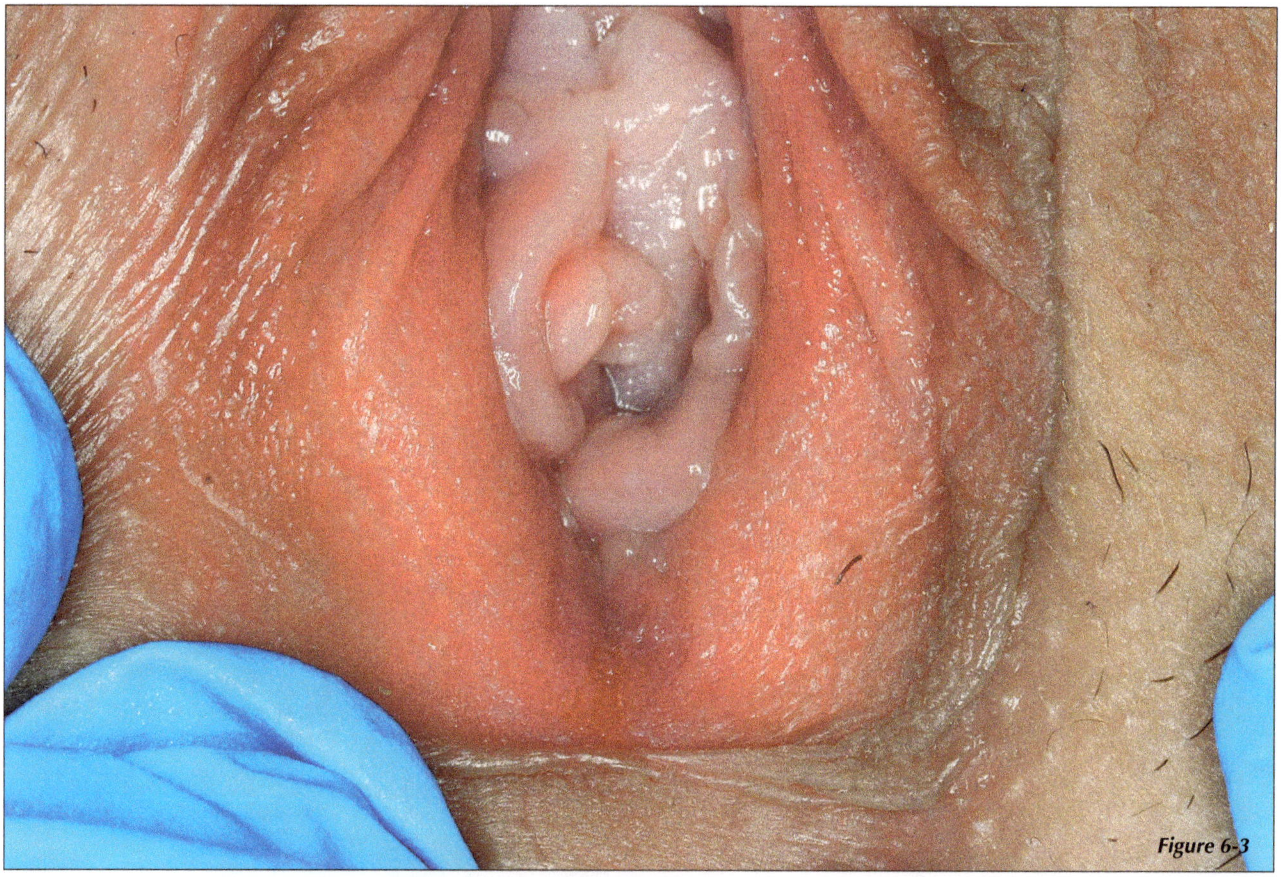

Figure 6-3

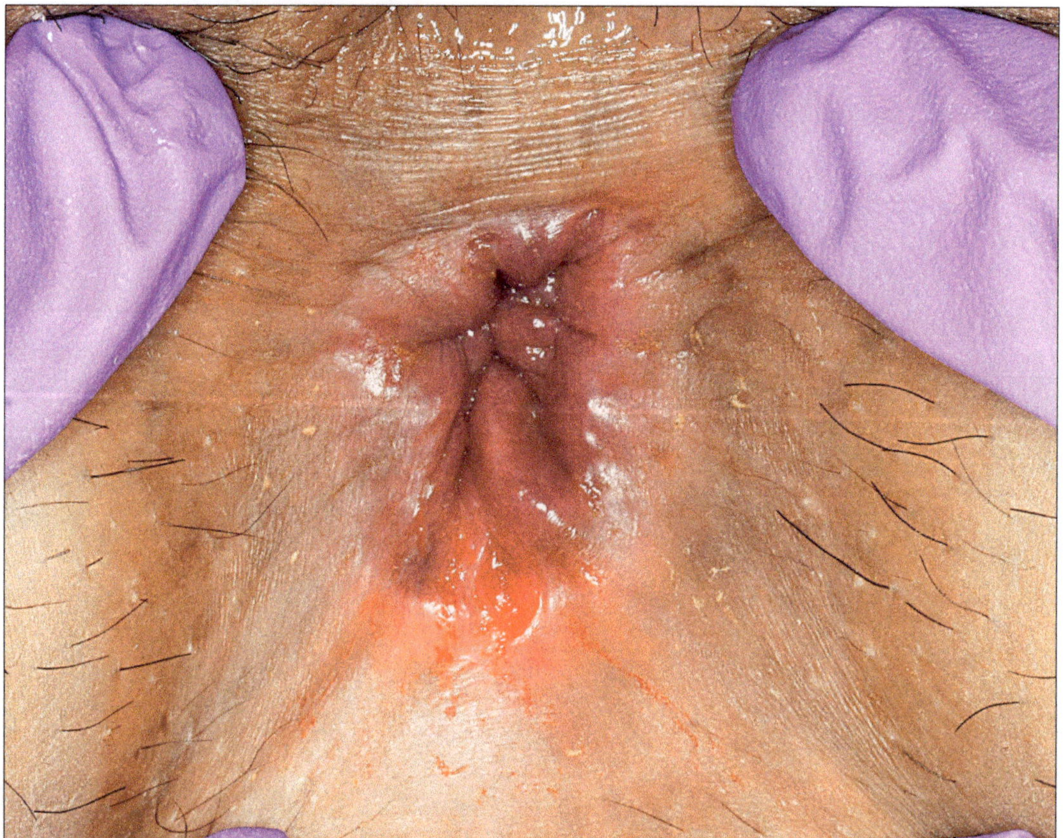

Figure 6-4

Activity 6-2. Injury Identification

Refer to **Figures 6-3** and **6-4**. Identify any injuries in respect to their anatomical location. Give objective descriptions when documenting findings.

Activity 6-3. Evidence Collection

Using the history and photographs provided, list the evidence you will collect from the patient. Please list the evidence in the order it will be collected.

Activity 6-4. Treatment

Describe the treatment you will offer the patient based on her history and your findings.

Chapter 7

Incapacitated Sexual Assault: 24-year-old Female Patient in a Psychiatric Facility

Objectives

After completing the exercises presented in this chapter, the student will be able to:

1. *Correctly identify the anogenital anatomy of a 24-year-old female patient.*
2. *Identify and document injuries based on an analysis of case photographs.*
3. *List at least 3 items of evidence that should be collected.*
4. *Discuss treatment options based on the patient's history.*

Case History

Emma, a 24-year-old woman, said she had been "working the streets" in downtown Los Angeles for about 2 years. She had been feeling increasingly depressed and last night attempted to take her own life. Emma's pimp found her unconscious in the hotel room and she was taken to the emergency department for treatment. After evaluation, Emma was admitted to a nearby psychiatric facility for a 72-hour hold, where she remained on suicide watch. After receiving her evening medications, she was assisted to her room. Due to the sedative effect of her medications, Emma was expected to sleep for several hours. The following morning, Emma told a nurse, "It hurts down there. I don't know what he did." Emma proceeded to say she thought the male aide snuck into her room and orally, vaginally, and anally penetrated her. The nursing staff, having recently received an in-service on sexual assault, immediately alerted their supervisor of Emma's concerns and placed her stained panties in a brown paper bag. Emma was taken by ambulance to the emergency department. The police accompanied the ambulance. When the forensic nurse interviewed Emma, she repeated several times that "it hurts" and pointed between her legs.

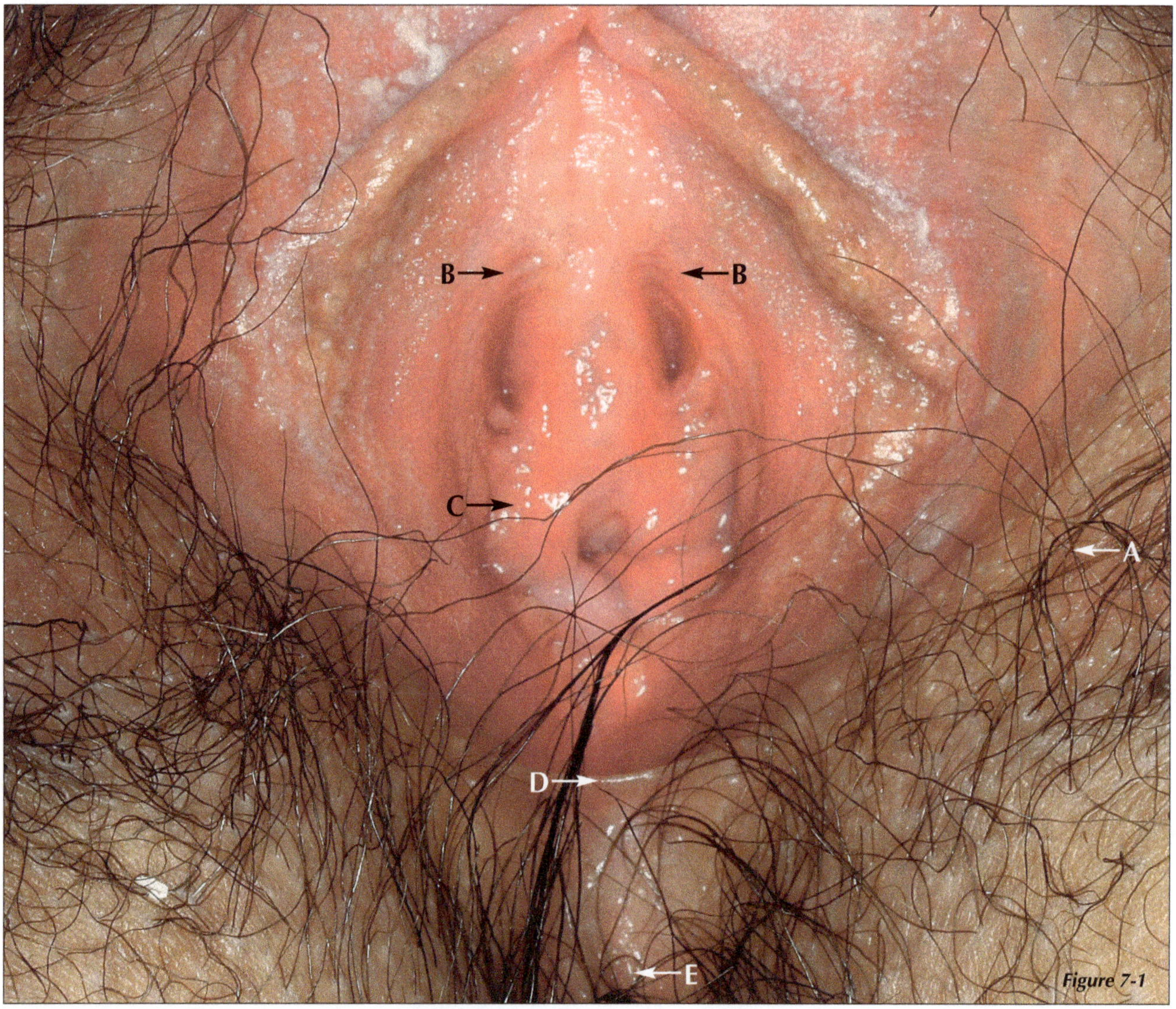

Figure 7-1

Anatomical Skills 7-1

Refer to **Figure 7-1**. Name the corresponding anatomical locations.

Arrow A: ____________________

Arrow B: ____________________

Arrow C: ____________________

Arrow D: ____________________

Arrow E: ____________________

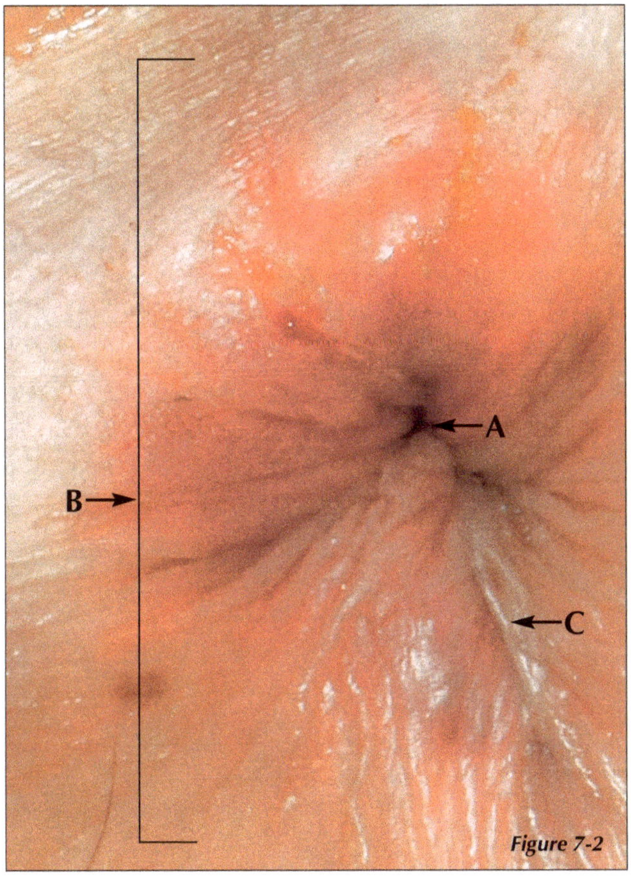

Anatomical Skills 7-2

Refer to **Figure 7-2**. Name the corresponding anatomical locations.

Arrow A: ______________________________

Arrow B: ______________________________

Arrow C: ______________________________

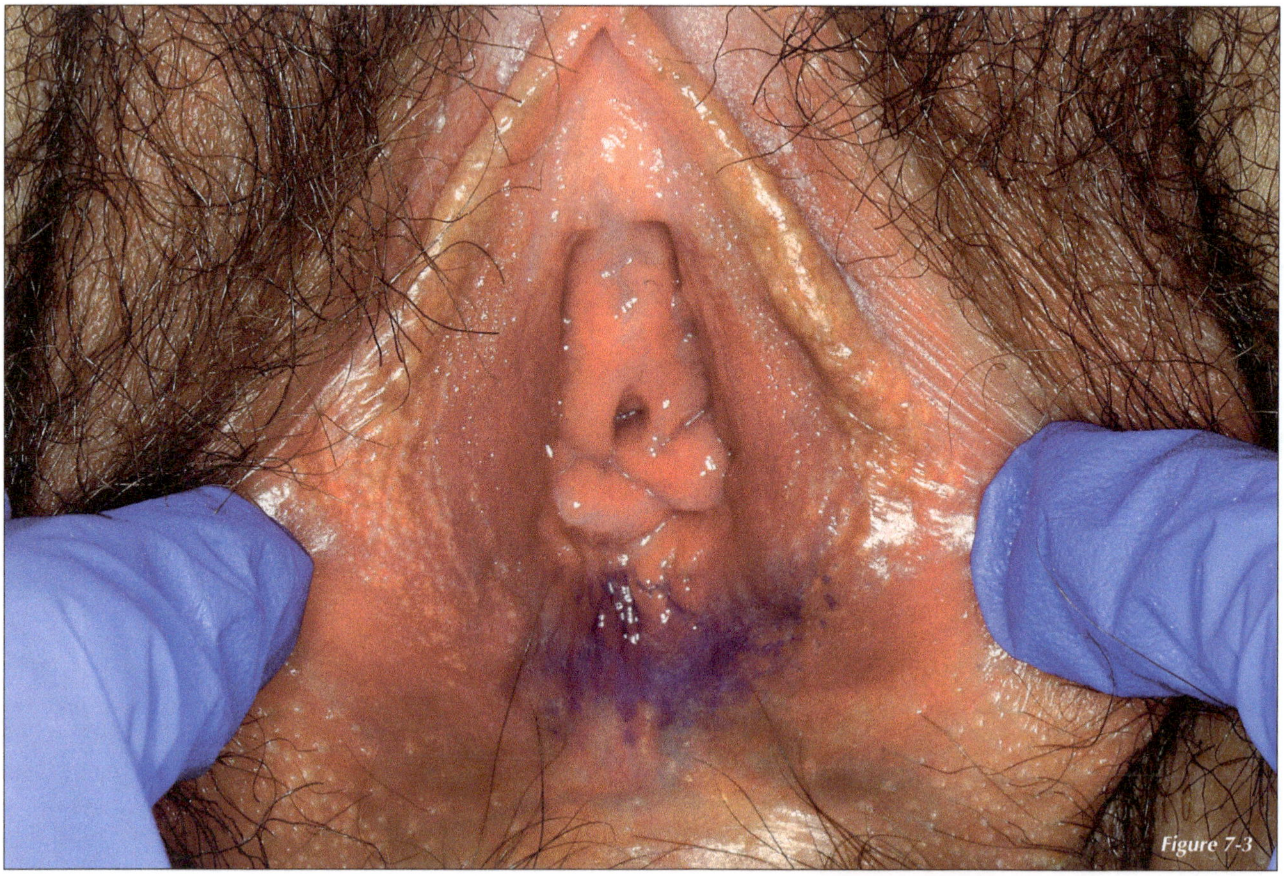

Figure 7-3

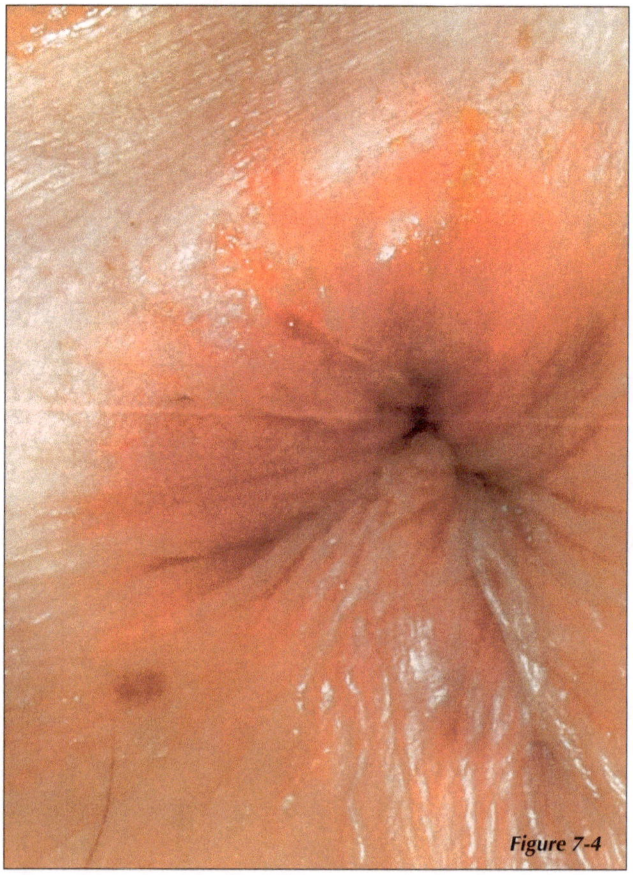

Figure 7-4

Activities 7-1, 7-2, and 7-3

Activity 7-1. Injury Identification

Refer to **Figures 7-3** and **7-4**. Identify any injuries in respect to their anatomical location. Give objective descriptions when documenting findings.

Activity 7-2. Evidence Collection

Using the history and photographs provided, list the evidence you will collect from the patient. Please list the evidence in the order it will be collected.

Activity 7-3. Treatment

Describe the treatment you will offer the patient based on her history and your findings.

Chapter 8

SEXUAL ASSAULT AND INTIMATE PARTNER VIOLENCE: 32-YEAR-OLD FEMALE PATIENT

OBJECTIVES

After completing the exercises presented in this chapter, the student will be able to:

1. *Correctly identify the anogenital anatomy of a 32-year-old female patient.*
2. *Identify and document injuries based on an analysis of case photographs.*
3. *List at least 3 items of evidence that should be collected.*
4. *Discuss treatment options based on the patient's history.*

CASE HISTORY

Mercedes is a 32-year-old woman who called the police to report an assault by her partner. During the law enforcement interview, she requested to go to the hospital because she was experiencing increasing stomach pain. Mercedes has been in a long-term relationship with a woman named Lisa, whom she describes as "sometimes violent." Mercedes said she was tired last night and when she rejected Lisa's sexual advances Lisa "became pushy and aggressive like she does sometimes." Mercedes described how Lisa tied her to the bed with handcuffs, repeatedly inserted a dildo vaginally and anally, and then performed cunnilingus on her. When Lisa finished she walked out of the room and left the apartment. Mercedes said, "I was so scared she wouldn't come back because when she left I was still handcuffed to the bed and couldn't call anyone for help. Finally, this morning, she came back and let me go. I acted like nothing happened, and she left me alone. I went to a coffee shop and called another friend, and she encouraged me to call the police." Lisa then told the forensic nurse, "It hurt really bad and there was blood on the sheets."

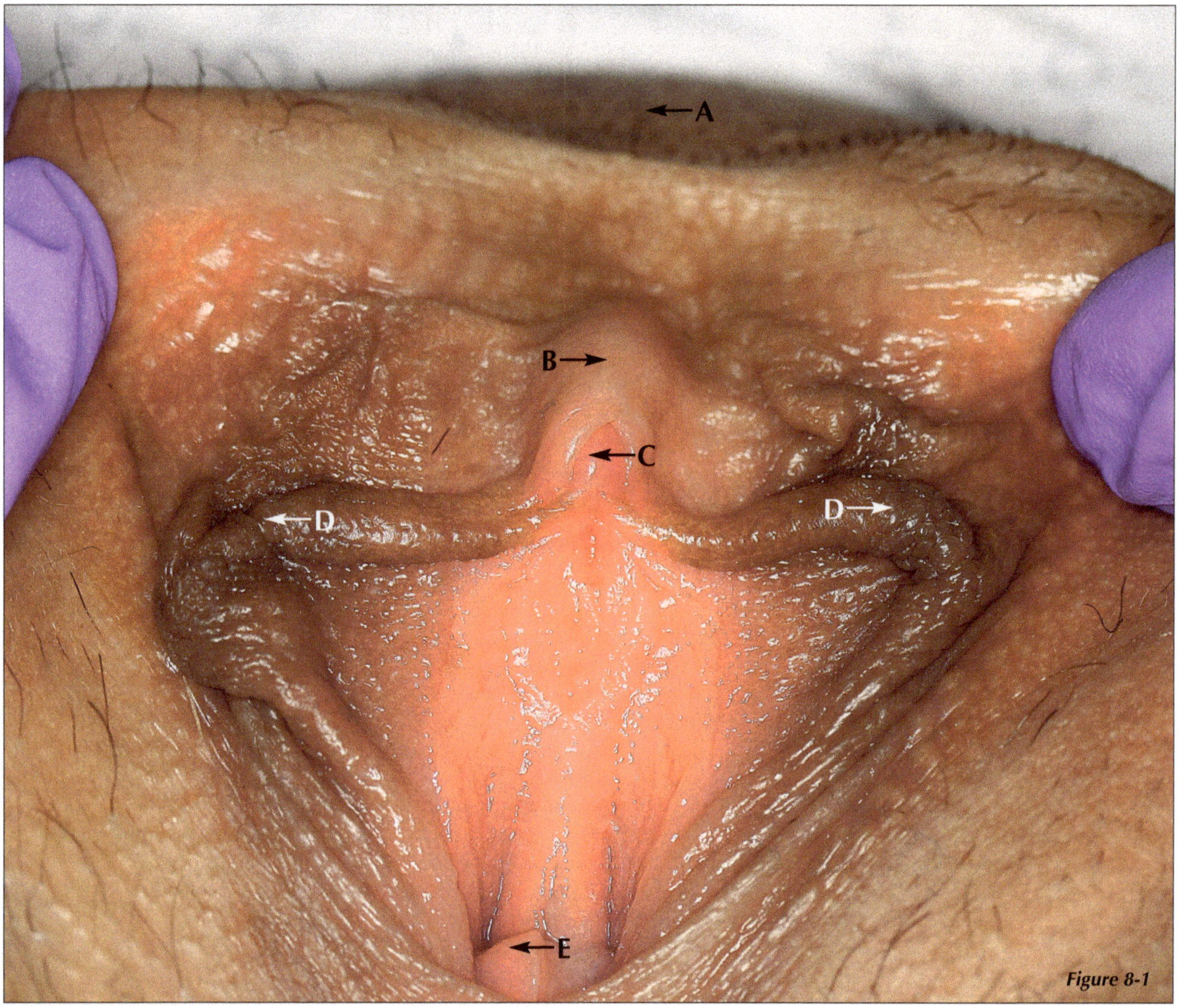

Figure 8-1

Anatomical Skills 8-1

Refer to **Figure 8-1**. Name the corresponding anatomical locations.

Arrow A: ____________________

Arrow B: ____________________

Arrow C: ____________________

Arrow D: ____________________

Arrow E: ____________________

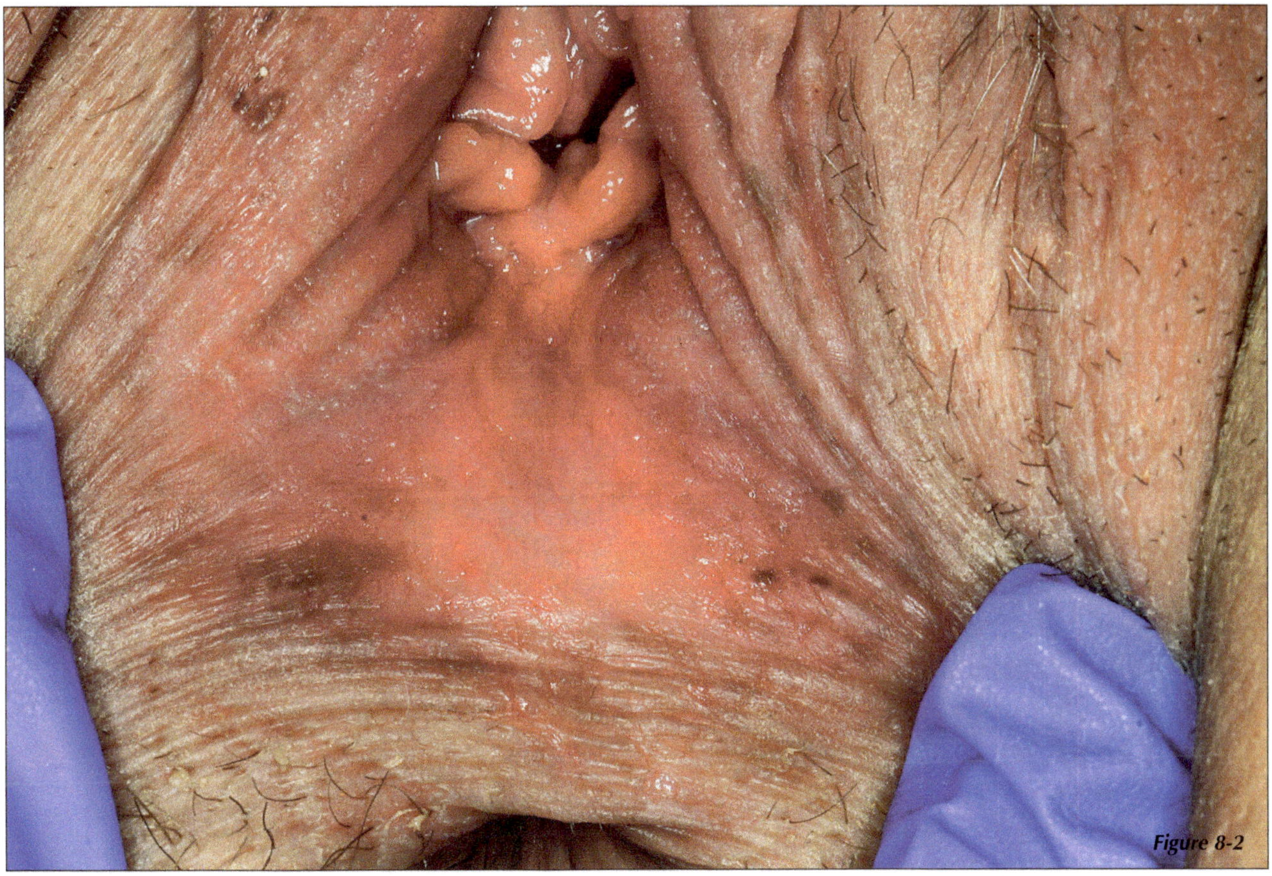

Figure 8-2

Activities 8-1, 8-2, and 8-3

Activity 8-1. Injury Identification

Refer to **Figures 8-2, 8-3,** and **8-4**. Identify any injuries in respect to their anatomical location. Give objective descriptions when documenting findings.

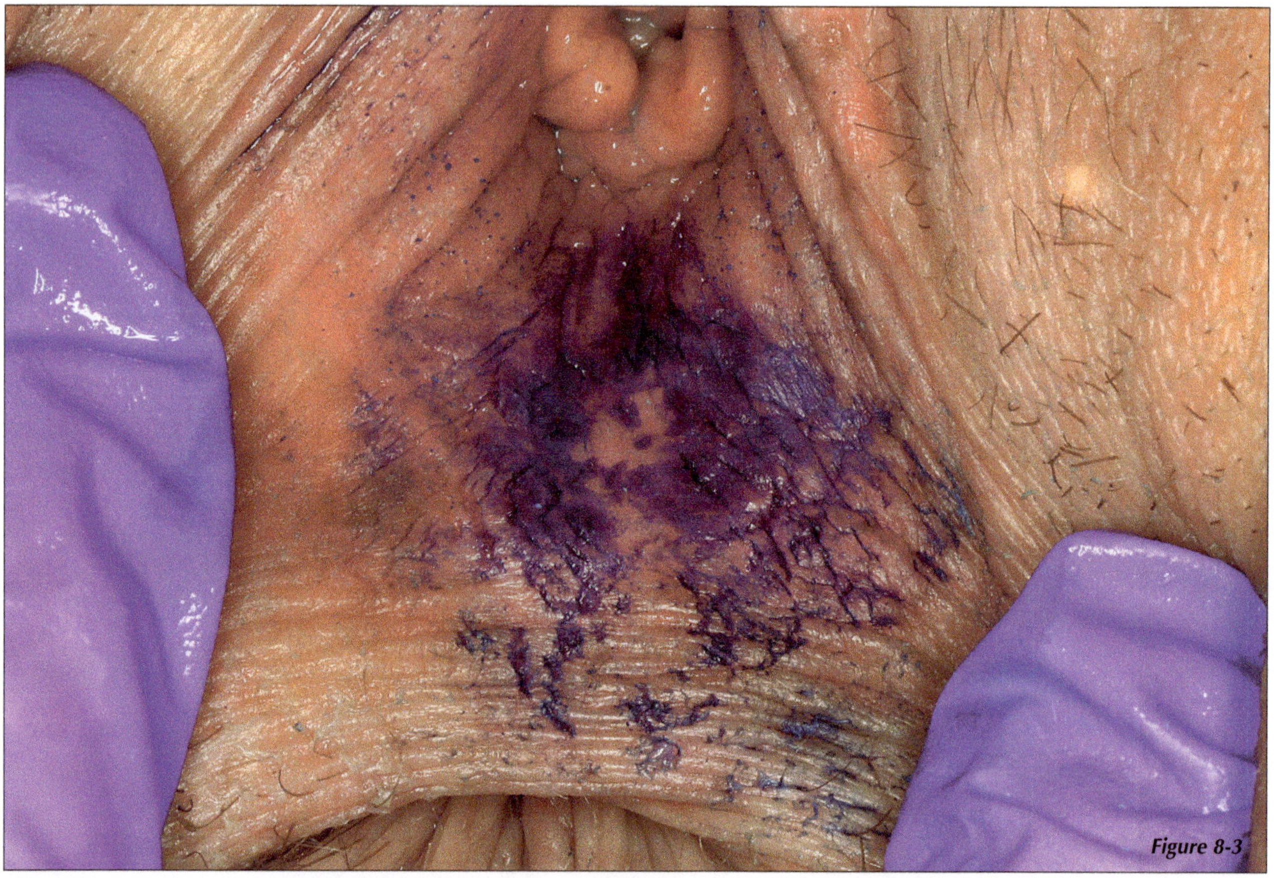

Figure 8-3

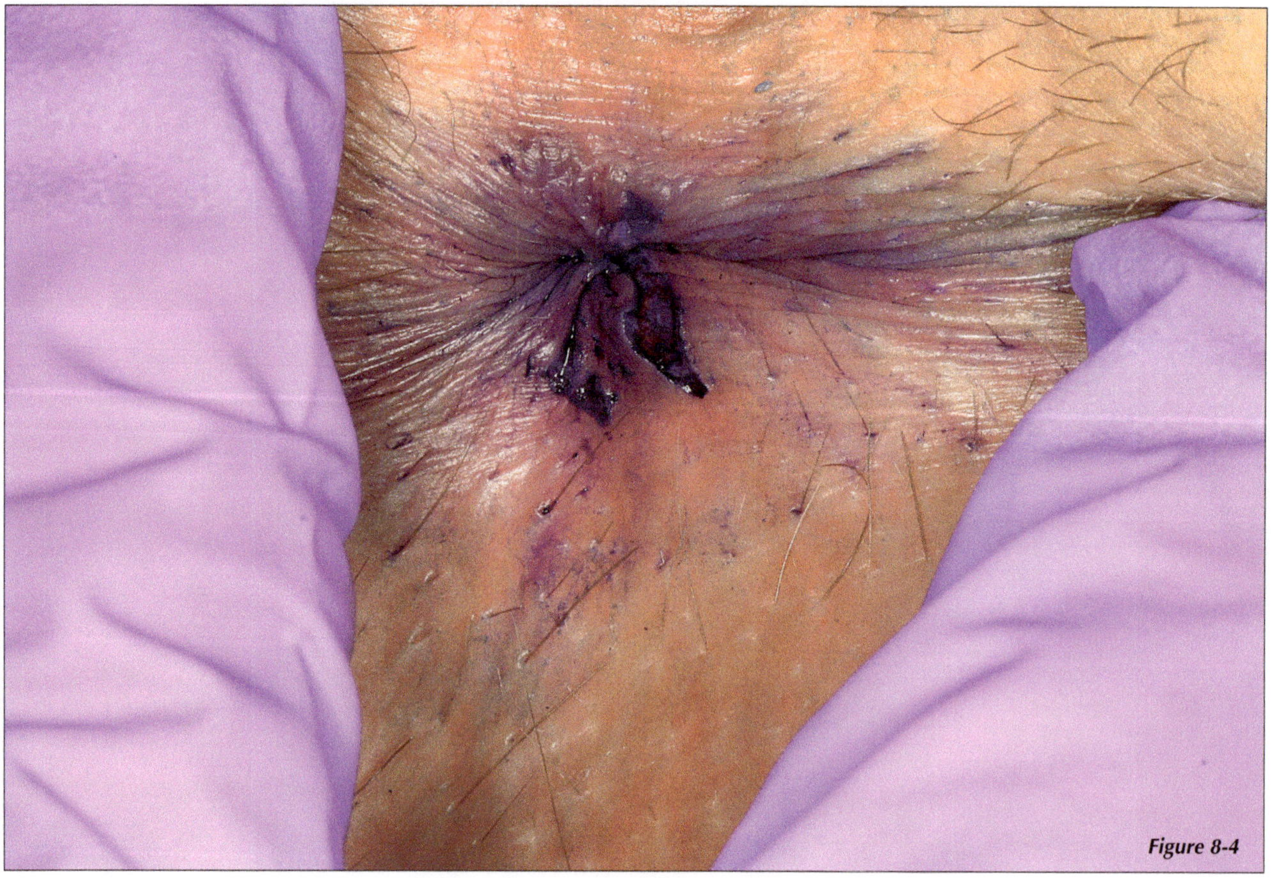

Figure 8-4

Activity 8-2. Evidence Collection

Using the history and photographs provided, list the evidence you will collect from the patient. Please list the evidence in the order it will be collected.

Activity 8-3. Treatment

Describe the treatment you will offer the patient based on her history and your findings.

NOTES

Chapter 9

Sexual Assault: 20-year-old Female Patient

Objectives

After completing the exercises presented in this chapter, the student will be able to:

1. *Correctly identify the anogenital anatomy of a 20-year-old female patient.*
2. *Identify and document injuries based on an analysis of case photographs.*
3. *List at least 3 items of evidence that should be collected.*
4. *Discuss treatment options based on the patient's history.*

Case History

Carol, a 20-year-old Marine, is home visiting her family and friends after being stationed in Iraq. Earlier tonight she went out to the movies with a group of friends. Jake, one of her friends, offers to give her a ride home. On the way home he pulls the car over in a secluded area not far from her house and tells her he is going to have sex with her. Carol is stunned and looks at him, not saying a word. When he doesn't say anything to her, she attempts to open the car door, but it is locked. He grabs her by the neck and puts her seat back. He climbs on top of her and pulls her pants down and her underwear to the side. At first he penetrates her vaginally with his fingers then proceeds to vaginally penetrate her with his penis. When he is done and moves back to the driver's seat, she pulls up her pants. Jake says, "I will call you tomorrow to see if you want to do anything" and then drops her off at her home. Carol calls a female friend and confides in her about what happened. Her friend listens to her story and tells Carol she was raped and should report the incident. Carol then calls the police and tells them what happened. They advise that she not void or change clothes, to go to the hospital, and they will meet her there. Carol tells the forensic nurse, "I didn't know what to do. I was so scared that he'd hurt me. I could tell by the look in his eyes he was someone else. That wasn't Jake; Jake wouldn't do that."

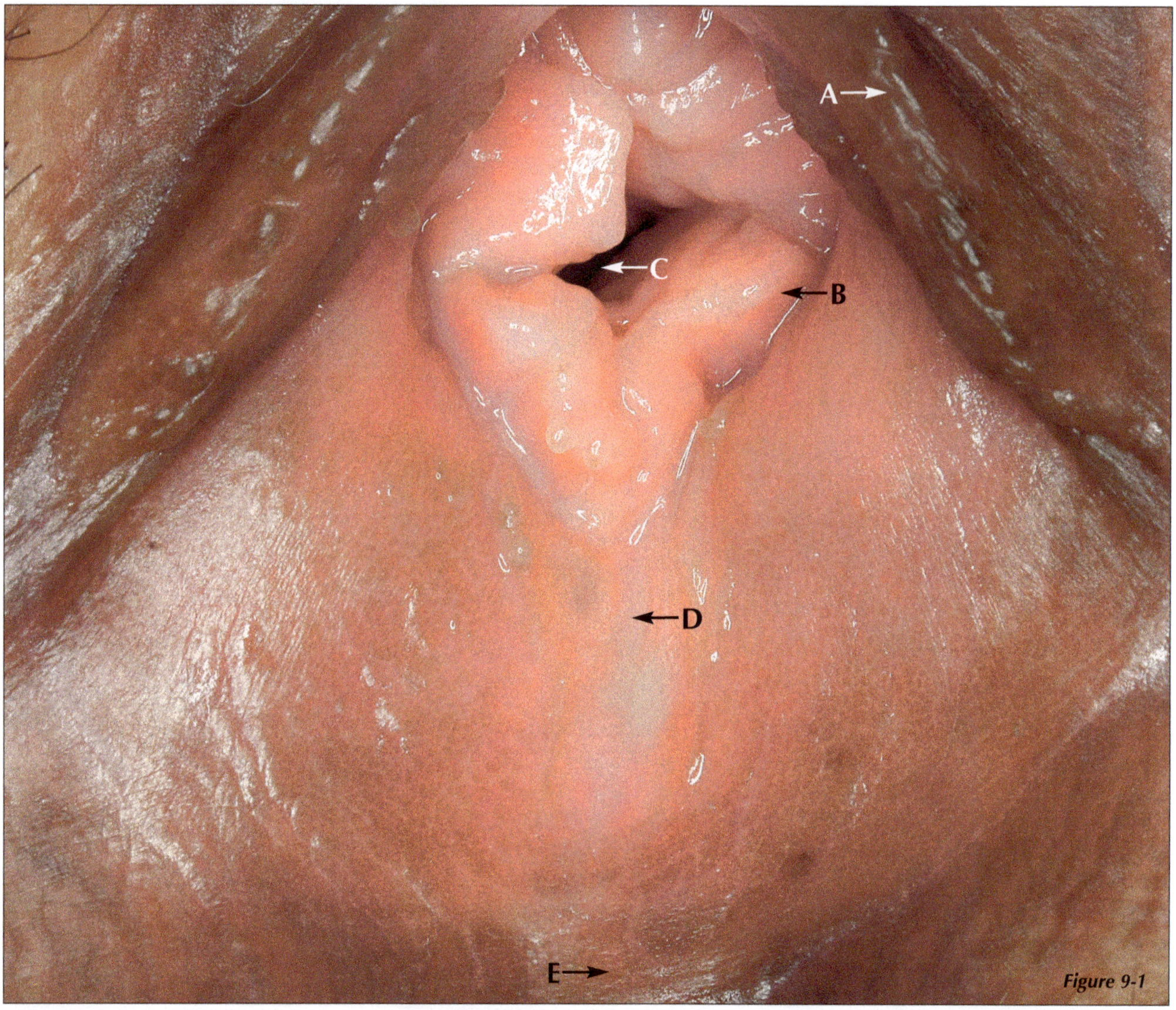

Figure 9-1

ANATOMICAL SKILLS 9-1

Refer to **Figure 9-1**. Name the corresponding anatomical locations.

Arrow A: ______________________________

Arrow B: ______________________________

Arrow C: ______________________________

Arrow D: ______________________________

Arrow E: ______________________________

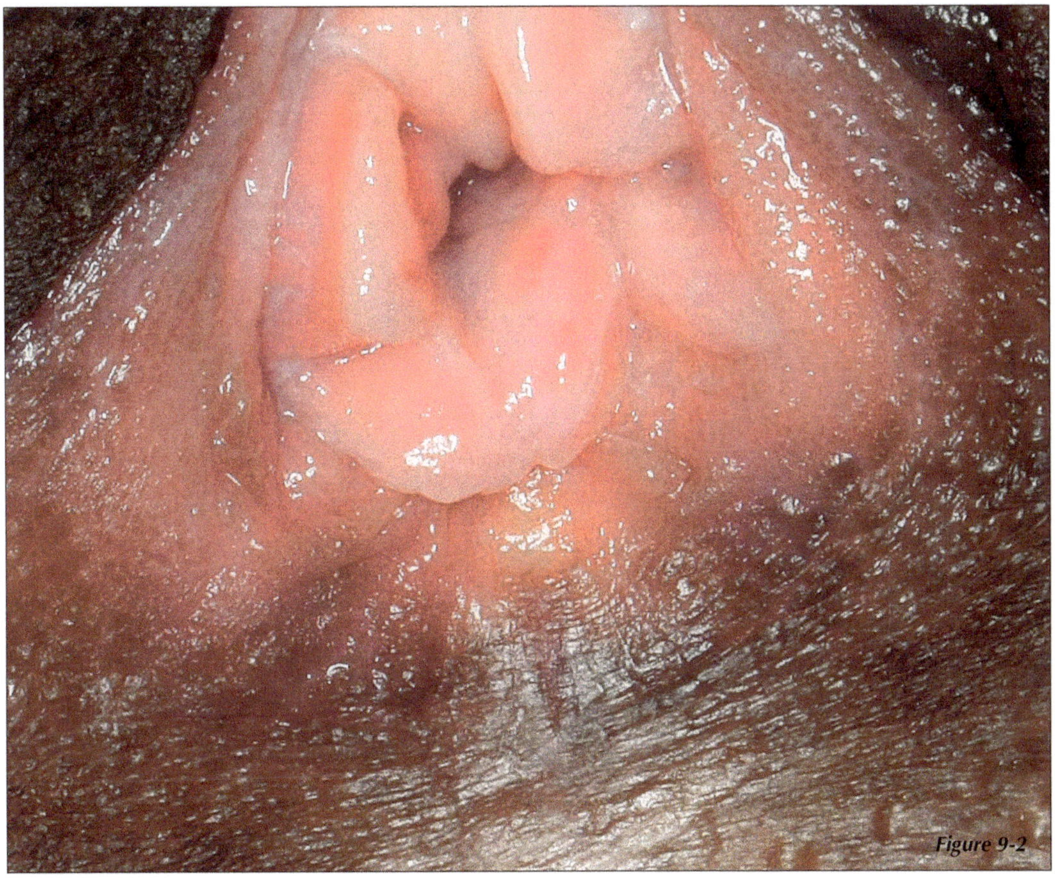

Figure 9-2

Activities 9-1, 9-2, and 9-3

Activity 9-1. Injury Identification

Refer to **Figure 9-2**. Identify any injuries in respect to their anatomical location. Give objective descriptions when documenting findings.

Activity 9-2. Evidence Collection

Using the history and photographs provided, list the evidence you will collect from the patient. Please list the evidence in the order it will be collected.

Activity 9-3. Treatment

Describe the treatment you will offer the patient based on her history and your findings.

Chapter 10

Documenting a History and Reviewing a Case

Objectives

After completing the exercises presented in this chapter, the student will be able to:

1. *Document the patient's history of assault.*
2. *Correctly identify the oral and/or anogenital anatomy presented in the case study.*
3. *Correctly label all injuries based on an analysis of the photographs.*
4. *State what evidence should be collected.*
5. *Devise a one-page treatment plan for the patient.*

Instructions

The purpose of the following exercise is to teach you and your colleagues how to conduct a peer review of cases in your program. Choose a case for review, document the patient's history, and collect photographs taken during the examination. Once a case has been selected, items documented, and photodocumentation is available for review, you and your colleagues will be able to proceed with the review as outlined here. Please note that you will need to document your responses on a separate piece of paper for this exercise.

Anatomical Skills 10-1

Review the photodocumentation and identify structures of the oral and/or anogenital anatomy. It will be helpful if the person presenting the case has marked and labeled these structures or area prior to the review.

Activities 10-1, 10-2, and 10-3

Activity 10-1. Injury Identification

Identify any injuries in respect to their anatomical location. Give objective descriptions when documenting findings.

Activity 10-2. Evidence Collection

Using the history and photographs you have assembled, list the evidence you will collect from the patient. Please list the evidence in the order it will be collected.

Activity 10-3. Treatment

Describe the treatment you will offer the patient based on his or her history and your findings.

Recommended Reading

Aiken MM. Documenting sexual abuse in prepubertal girls. *Am J Maternal Child Nurs.* 1990;15(3):176-177.

Ambuel B, Trent K, Lenahan P, et al. *Competencies Needed by Health Professionals for Addressing Exposure to Violence and Abuse in Patient Care.* Eden Prairie, MN: Academy on Violence and Abuse; 2011.

American Medical Association. Competencies necessary for physicians to provide quality care to victims of family and intimate partner violence and abuse. Paper presented at: American Medical Association National Advisory Council on Violence and Abuse; 2006; Chicago, IL; unpublished manuscript.

Block RW, Ismailji T, Schneider F, Dolezal T. Creating core competencies for health education on violence and abuse. Presented at: Preconference Institute, Family Violence Prevention Fund Conference on Violence and Health; October 8, 2009; New Orleans, LA.

Boehm H, Bonnel W. The use of peer review in nursing education and clinical practice. *J Nurses Staff Dev.* 2010;26(3):108-115.

Centers for Disease Control and Prevention. Sexually Transmitted Diseases Treatment Guidelines, 2010. http://www.cdc.gov/std/treatment/2010/sexual-assault.htm. Updated January 28, 2011.

Department of Health. Protocol for the Acute Care of the Adult Patient Reporting Sexual Assault. http://www.health.state.ny.us/professionals/protocols_and_guidelines/sexual_assault. Revised October 2008.

DNA Initiative. Evidence Collection and Preservation. http://www.dna.gov/audiences/investigators/know/collection.

Ferguson CT, Faugno D. The SAFE CARE model: maintaining competency in sexual assault examinations utilizing patient simulation methods. *J Forensic Nurs.* 2009;5(2):109-114.

Girardin B, Faugno D, Spencer M, Giardino A. *Sexual Assault: Victimization Across the Lifespan: A Color Atlas.* St. Louis, MO: GW Medical Inc; 2003. *Sexual Assault: Victimization Across the Lifespan: A Clinical Guide and Color Atlas*; vol 2.

Ledray LE, Burgess AW, Giardino AP. *Medical Response to Adult Sexual Assault: A Resource for Clinicians and Related Professionals.* St. Louis, MO: STM Learning Inc; 2011.

Morgan JA. Comparison of cervical os versus vaginal evidentiary findings during sexual assault exam. *J Emerg Nurs.* 2008;34(2):102-105.

Muram D. Child sexual abuse: relationship between sexual acts and genital findings. *Child Abuse Negl.* 1989;13(2):211-216.

New York State Division of Criminal Justice Services. Appendix Q. http://www.health.state.ny.us/professionals/protocols_and_guidelines/sexual_assault/docs/protocol_appendix_q.pdf. Published October 1, 2008.

Office of the Attorney General. Texas Evidence Collection Protocol. https://www.oag.state.tx.us/AG_Publications/pdfs/evidence_collection.pdf. Published 1998.

US Department of Justice Office on Violence Against Women. A National Protocol for Sexual Assault Medical Forensic Examinations. http://samfe.dna.gov. Published September 2004.

US Department of Justice Office on Violence Against Women. A National Protocol for Sexual Assault Medical Forensic Examinations Adult/Adolescents. https://www.ncjrs.gov/pdffiles1/ovw/206554.pdf. Published September 2004.

Wood D. Peer review opportunities to improve nursing care. NurseZone Web site. http://www.nursezone.com/Nursing-News-Events/more-features/Peer-Review-Offers-Opportunities-to-Improve-Nursing-Care_29908.aspx. Published 2009.

Answer Key

Note to students

Community standards and agency protocols for evidence collection, prophylactic treatment, patient referrals, and follow-up vary across the United States and internationally. It is the student's responsibility to know his or her community standards and agency protocols AND the rationale surrounding any variations where national or international standards or recommendations exist.

When documenting findings in the medical forensic record, documentation should include approximate length, width, shape, and color of injuries. This level of documentation is not possible when reviewing photodocumentation as presented in these case studies. Limitations to assessment of injury via photodocumentation are related to several variables, including scale, angle, lighting, equipment settings, picture quality, and provider technique (eg, separation, traction).

The case studies in this book are brief summaries of complex patient encounters. The figures provided with each case study represent a sample of the photodocumentation collected during the medical forensic examination. Please note the detail and extent of evidence collection, prophylactic treatment, patient referrals, and recommended follow-up are based on these brief summaries, not on the additional details that would be available during an actual patient encounter. Also, the authors of the *SANE/SAFE Forensic Learning Series* purposefully created the answer key for a broad audience to reflect the diversity and scope of practice of individuals completing this book. In doing so, it is recognized that the answer key may often reflect those roles that have a more limited scope of practice (eg, RN versus APRN or MD).

Chapter 1: Sexual Assault: 41-year-old Female Patient with Down's Syndrome

Anatomical Skills 1-1

A. Right labia minora

B. Right labia majora

C. Hymen

D. Fossa navicularis

E. Posterior fourchette

Activity 1-1. Injury Identification

— Vestibule/fossa navicularis: Abrasion from 3 to 10 o'clock with positive dye uptake (**Figure 1-2**)

— Hymen: Focal redness from 3 to 4 o'clock (**Figure 1-3**)

Activity 1-2. Evidence Collection

1. Photodocumentation: In many communities, photodocumentation will also be used as evidence in the investigative and judicial processes. Photodocumentation should occur throughout the medical forensic examination/evaluation and may include the following:

   — Patient upon initial presentation

   — Anterior and posterior hands

   — Foreign debris or substances on patient or clothing

   — Injuries

2. Clothing: Collect clothing; if applicable, collect second pair of underwear worn.

- If clothing changed prior to arrival, notify law enforcement that original items of clothing are not with patient.

3. Alternate Light Source: If community standard, examine patient with Wood's Lamp/ALS.
   - NOTE: Collect specimens from all areas based on history regardless if negative or positive fluorescence PLUS any areas of positive fluorescence.
4. Oral specimens: When history includes oral assault or is unknown for oral assault, consider collecting oral specimens as soon as possible and allowing patient to complete oral hygiene.
   - Collect specimens from lips, around mouth, and corners of mouth.
   - Collect specimens from oral cavity.
   - NOTE: These are NOT buccal swabs for DNA standard. Specimens collected for evidence and buccal swabs for DNA standard are collected from different anatomical locations. Additionally, there should be an oral-hygiene protocol between collection of specimens for evidence and collection of buccal swabs for DNA standard. Document oral hygiene in medical forensic record.
5. Anogenital specimens:
   - NOTE: Order of specimen collection varies depending on community standards and agency protocols.
   - Collect hair present from vaginal introitus (**Figure 1-2**).
   - Collect vulvar specimens.
   - If practice includes use of Toluidine Blue Dye, apply and assess for injury.
   - Insert speculum and collect specimens from vaginal vault and cervical os.
     - NOTE: If used, document use of lubrication on medical forensic record.
   - Collect specimens from perianal skin, anus, and rectum.
     - NOTE: If practice includes use of anoscope, collect specimens from tissue distal to the tip of anoscope; type of lubrication used should be documented in the medical forensic record.
   - If drainage observed from any genital orifice, collect specimen of drainage
6. Collect blood and toxicology screens per community standard or agency protocol.
7. DNA standard: Method and time of collection will vary based on community standards and agency protocols.
   - If practice is to collect buccal specimens for DNA standard, this may be completed following oral assessment or at the end of the exam if history does not warrant assessment of the oral cavity.
   - If practice is to collect blood specimens for DNA standard (eg, blood standard card, tube of blood), this may be completed when other lab specimens are collected; if other lab specimens are not collected during the exam, this may be completed at end of the exam.
8. If patient must urinate prior to exam, give 4x4 gauze pad to wipe vulva prior to urination and another 4x4 gauze pad to wipe vulva following urination. Collect both 4x4 gauze pads and add these items to the evidence kit.

Activity 1-3. Treatment

- If applicable or desired by patient, offer pregnancy testing and Emergency Hormonal Contraception and provide related patient education.
- Recommend and/or provide medications based on Centers for Disease Control (CDC) guidelines or local/community protocol and provide related patient education.
- Offer STI screenings including HIV screening, referral, and post-exposure prophylaxis (PEP) per CDC guidelines or local/community protocols and provide related patient education.
- Refer for counseling services via rape crisis center, advocacy program, or other local service provider or counseling center.

— Refer to Victim Witness program for assistance with medical expenses not related to the medical forensic examination.

— Provide discharge instructions for care of injury, including a reminder of the presence of Toluidine Blue Dye, and provide anticipatory guidance based on patient history, verbal/nonverbal communication during examination, and patient questions.

Chapter 2: Sexual Assault: 32-year-old Male Patient

Anatomical Skills 2-1

A. Shaft of penis

B. Corona of glans penis

C. Glans of penis

D. Scrotum

Anatomical Skills 2-2

A. Perineum

B. Anus

C. Perianal skin folds

D. Perianal venous engorgement

Activity 2-1. Injury Identification

— Anus: Laceration at 1 o'clock extending onto anal verge (**Figure 2-3**); active bleeding upon manipulation (**Figure 2-4**)

—NOTE: Consider direction of drainage from site of bleeding. When traction released, there is skin-to-skin contact resulting in the blood appearing on perianal skin from 4 to 7 o'clock.

Activity 2-2. Evidence Collection

1. Photodocumentation: In many communities, photodocumentation will also be used as evidence in the investigative and judicial processes. Photodocumentation should occur throughout the medical forensic examination/evaluation and may include the following:

   — Patient upon initial presentation

   — Anterior and posterior hands

   — Foreign debris or substances on patient or clothing

   — Injuries

2. Clothing: Collect clothing; if applicable, collect second pair of underwear worn.

   — If clothing changed prior to arrival and law enforcement is involved, notify law enforcement that original items of clothing are not with patient.

3. Collect washcloth patient used to stop the bleeding.

4. Alternate Light Source: If community standard, examine patient with Wood's Lamp/ALS.

   — NOTE: Collect specimens from all areas based on history regardless if negative or positive fluorescence PLUS any areas of positive fluorescence.

5. Oral specimens: When history includes oral assault or is unknown for oral assault, consider collecting oral specimens as soon as possible and allowing patient to complete oral hygiene.

   — Collect specimens from lips, around mouth, and corners of mouth.

   — Collect specimens from oral cavity.

   — NOTE: These are NOT buccal swabs for DNA standard. Specimens collected for evidence and buccal swabs for DNA standard are collected from different anatomical locations. Additionally, there should be an oral hygiene protocol between collection of specimens for evidence and collection of buccal swabs for DNA standard. Document oral hygiene in medical forensic record.

6. Anogenital specimens:
   - Collect specimens from penis, corona, frenulum, and base of penis.
   - Collect specimens from scrotal area adjacent to penis.
   - Collect specimens from perianal skin, anus, and rectum; if anal dilation occurs, swab rectum if possible, taking care to avoid blood fluids to prevent dilution of the sample.
   - NOTE: If practice includes use of anoscope, collect specimens from tissue distal to the tip of anoscope; type of lubrication used should be documented in the medical forensic record.
7. Collect blood and toxicology screens per community standard or agency protocol. If history includes concern for drug-facilitated sexual assault, collect blood and urine as soon as possible.
8. DNA standard: Method and time of collection will vary based on community standards and agency protocols.
   - If practice is to collect buccal specimens for DNA standard, this may be completed following oral assessment or at the end of the exam if history does not warrant assessment of the oral cavity.
   - If practice is to collect blood specimens for DNA standard (eg, blood standard card, tube of blood), this may be completed when other lab specimens are collected; if other lab specimens are not collected during the exam, this may be completed at end of the exam.

Activity 2-3. Treatment

- Recommend patient see emergency department provider (eg, MD, NP, PA) for evaluation of actively bleeding ano-rectal laceration.
- Recommend and/or provide medications based on Centers for Disease Control (CDC) guidelines or local/community protocol and provide related patient education.
- Offer STI screenings including HIV screening, referral, and post-exposure prophylaxis (PEP) per CDC guidelines or local/community protocols and provide related patient education.
- Refer for counseling services via rape crisis center, advocacy program, or other local service provider or counseling center.
- Refer to Victim Witness program for assistance with medical expenses not related to the medical forensic examination.
- Provide discharge instructions for care of injury and recommended follow-up and anticipatory guidance based on patient history, verbal/nonverbal communication during examination, and patient questions.

Chapter 3: Incapacitated Sexual Assault: 24-year-old Female Patient

Anatomical Skills 3-1

A. Urethral meatus

B. Vaginal introitus

C. Hymen

D. Fossa navicularis

E. Vaginal vestibule

Anatomical Skills 3-2

A. Anterior cervix

B. Cervical os

C. Left vaginal wall rugae

D. Posterior cervix

E. Posterior vaginal fornix

Anatomical Skills 3-3

A. Perineum

B. Anus

C. Perianal skin folds

D. Perianal venous engorgement

Activity 3-1. Injury Identification

— Vaginal vestibule: Generalized vestibular redness (**Figure 3-4**)

— Fossa navicularis: Abrasion from 4 to 7 o'clock with positive dye uptake (**Figure 3-4**)

— Posterior fourchette: Laceration extending onto fossa navicularis at 6 o'clock with positive dye uptake (**Figure 3-4**)

Activity 3-2. Injury Identification

— No visible injury (**Figure 3-5**)

Activity 3-3. Injury Identification

— Perianal tissue/anus: Perianal swelling from 4 to 7 o'clock extending onto anal verge; multiple lacerations from 5 to 7 o'clock and 11 to 12 o'clock; strands of mucoid-like substance bridging across anal opening (**Figure 3-6**).

Activity 3-4. Evidence Collection

1. Photodocumentation: In many communities, photodocumentation will also be used as evidence in the investigative and judicial processes. Photodocumentation should occur throughout the medical forensic examination/evaluation and may include the following:

   — Patient upon initial presentation

   — Anterior and posterior hands

   — Foreign debris or substances on patient or clothing

   — Injuries

2. Clothing: Collect clothing; if applicable, collect second pair of underwear worn.

   — If clothing changed prior to arrival and law enforcement is involved, notify law enforcement that original items of clothing are not with patient.

3. Alternate Light Source: If community standard, examine patient with Wood's Lamp/ALS.

   — NOTE: Collect specimens from all areas based on history regardless if negative or positive fluorescence PLUS any areas of positive fluorescence.

4. Oral specimens: When history includes oral assault or is unknown for oral assault, consider collecting oral specimens as soon as possible and allowing patient to complete oral hygiene.

   — Collect specimens from lips, around mouth, and corners of mouth.

   — Collect specimens from oral cavity.

   — NOTE: These are NOT buccal swabs for DNA standard. Specimens collected for evidence and buccal swabs for DNA standard are collected from different anatomical locations. Additionally, there should be an oral hygiene protocol between collection of specimens for evidence and collection of buccal swabs for DNA standard. Document oral hygiene in medical forensic record.

5. Collect specimens from both sides of neck.

6. Collect specimens from both breasts.

7. Anogenital specimens:

   — NOTE: Order of specimen collection varies depending on community standards and agency protocols.

— Collect vulvar specimens.

— If practice includes use of Toluidine Blue Dye, apply and assess for injury.

— Insert speculum and collect specimens from vaginal vault and cervical os.

— NOTE: If used, document use of lubrication on medical forensic record.

— Collect specimens from perianal skin, anus, and rectum.

— NOTE: If practice includes use of anoscope, collect specimens from tissue distal to the tip of anoscope; type of lubrication used should be documented in the medical forensic record.

— If drainage observed from any genital orifice, collect specimen of drainage.

8. Collect blood and toxicology screens per community standard or agency protocol. If history includes concern for drug-facilitated sexual assault, collect blood and urine as soon as possible.

9. DNA standard: Method and time of collection will vary based on community standards and agency protocols.

   — If practice is to collect buccal specimens for DNA standard, this may be completed following oral assessment or at the end of the exam if history does not warrant assessment of the oral cavity.

   — If practice is to collect blood specimens for DNA standard (eg, blood standard card, tube of blood), this may be completed when other lab specimens are collected; if other lab specimens are not collected during the exam, this may be completed at end of the exam.

10. If patient must urinate prior to exam, give 4x4 gauze pad to wipe vulva prior to urination and another 4x4 gauze pad to wipe vulva following urination. Collect both 4x4 gauze pads and add these items to the evidence kit.

Activity 3-5 Treatment

— If applicable or desired by patient, offer pregnancy testing and Emergency Hormonal Contraception and provide related patient education.

— Recommend and/or provide medications based on Centers for Disease Control (CDC) guidelines or local/community protocol and provide related patient education.

— Offer STI screenings including HIV screening, referral, and post-exposure prophylaxis (PEP) per CDC guidelines or local/community protocols and provide related patient education.

— Refer for counseling services via rape crisis center, advocacy program, or other local service provider or counseling center.

— Refer to Victim Witness program for assistance with medical expenses not related to the medical forensic examination.

— Provide discharge instructions for care of injury, including a reminder of the presence of Toluidine Blue Dye, and provide anticipatory guidance based on patient history, verbal/nonverbal communication during examination, and patient questions.

Chapter 4: Sexual Assault: 21-year-old Female College Student

Anatomical Skills 4-1

A. Clitoral hood

B. Right and left labia minora

C. Hymen

D. Fossa navicularis

E. Posterior fourchette

Anatomical Skills 4-2

A. Soft palate

B. Right palatopharyngeal arch

C. Posterior oropharynx

D. Right and left palatoglossal arch

E. Tongue

Activity 4-1. Injury Identification

— Palatoglossal arch: Bilateral redness and injection extending onto to soft palate (**Figure 4-3**)

— Uvula: Multiple petechiae (**Figure 4-3**)

— Palatopharyngeal arch: Bilateral redness and injection (**Figure 4-3**)

— Posterior oropharynx: Generalized redness and inflammation (**Figure 4-3**)

— Fossa navicularis: Abrasion from 4 to 8 o'clock (**Figure 4-4**)

Activity 4-2. Evidence Collection

1. Photodocumentation: In many communities, photodocumentation will also be used as evidence in the investigative and judicial processes. Photodocumentation should occur throughout the medical forensic examination/evaluation and may include the following:

   — Patient upon initial presentation

   — Anterior and posterior hands

   — Foreign debris or substances on patient or clothing

   — Injuries

2. Clothing: Collect clothing; if applicable, collect second pair of underwear worn.

   — If clothing changed prior to arrival and law enforcement is involved, notify law enforcement that original items of clothing are not with patient.

3. Alternate Light Source: If community standard, examine patient with Wood's Lamp/ALS.

   — NOTE: Collect specimens from all areas based on history regardless if negative or positive fluorescence PLUS any areas of positive fluorescence.

4. Oral specimens: When history includes oral assault or is unknown for oral assault, consider collecting oral specimens as soon as possible and allowing patient to complete oral hygiene.

   — Collect specimens from lips, around mouth, and corners of mouth.

   — Collect specimens from oral cavity.

   — NOTE: These are NOT buccal swabs for DNA standard. Specimens collected for evidence and buccal swabs for DNA standard are collected from different anatomical locations. Additionally, there should be an oral hygiene protocol between collection of specimens for evidence and collection of buccal swabs for DNA standard. Document oral hygiene in medical forensic record.

5. Anogenital specimens:

   — Collect vulvar specimens.

   — If practice includes use of Toluidine Blue Dye, apply and assess for injury.

   — Insert speculum and collect specimens from vaginal vault and cervical os.

      — NOTE: If used, document use of lubrication on medical forensic record.

   — If drainage observed from any genital orifice, collect specimen of drainage.

6. Collect blood and toxicology screens per community standard or agency protocol.
7. DNA standard: Method and time of collection will vary based on community standards and agency protocols.
   - If practice is to collect buccal specimens for DNA standard, this may be completed following oral assessment or at the end of the exam if history does not warrant assessment of the oral cavity.
   - If practice is to collect blood specimens for DNA standard (eg, blood standard card, tube of blood), this may be completed when other lab specimens are collected; if other lab specimens are not collected during the exam, this may be completed at the end of the exam.
8. If patient must urinate prior to exam, give 4x4 gauze pad to wipe vulva prior to urination and another 4x4 gauze pad to wipe vulva following urination. Collect both 4x4 gauze pads and add these items to the evidence kit.
9. Patient vomited on floor of apartment bathroom following an oral assault with ejaculation. If law enforcement is involved, inform of emesis and potential of ejaculate present in emesis.

Activity 4-3. Treatment

- If applicable or desired by patient, offer pregnancy testing and Emergency Hormonal Contraception and provide related patient education.
- Recommend and/or provide medications based on Centers for Disease Control (CDC) guidelines or local/community protocol and provide related patient education.
- Offer STI screenings including HIV screening, referral, and post-exposure prophylaxis (PEP) per CDC guidelines or local/community protocols and provide related patient education.
- Refer for counseling services via rape crisis center, advocacy program, or other local service provider or counseling center.
- Refer to Victim Witness program for assistance with medical expenses not related to the medical forensic examination.
- Provide discharge instructions for care of injury, including a reminder of the presence of Toluidine Blue Dye, and provide anticipatory guidance based on patient history, verbal/nonverbal communication during examination, and patient questions.

Chapter 5: Drug-Facilitated Sexual Assault: 15-year-old Female Patient

Anatomical Skills 5-1

A. Periurethral tissue

B. Hymen

C. Vaginal introitus

D. Fossa navicularis

E. Posterior fourchette

Anatomical Skills 5-2

A. Cervix/posterior cervix

B. Sqaumocolumnar junction

C. Left labia majora

D. Cervical os

Activity 5-1. Injury Identification

- Posterior fourchette: Abrasion with positive dye uptake (student will be unable to identify margins of abrasion using clock terminology [eg, from 4 to 8 o'clock] due to angle of traction) (**Figure 5-3**)

— Vestibule/Fossa navicularis: Vestibular redness from 3 to 9 o'clock extending on to perihymenal tissue (**Figure 5-3**)

— Hymen: Focal redness at 3 o'clock (**Figure 5-3**)

— Cervix: Multiple petechiae circumferentially around cervical os (**Figure 5-4**)

— NOTE: This may be a normal variant for this patient; follow-up evaluation is needed to determine if normal variant.

Activity 5-2. Evidence Collection

1. Photodocumentation: In many communities, photodocumentation will also be used as evidence in the investigative and judicial processes. Photodocumentation should occur throughout the medical forensic examination/evaluation and may include the following:

   — Patient upon initial presentation

   — Anterior and posterior hands

   — Foreign debris or substances on patient or clothing

   — Injuries

2. Clothing: Patient was found naked and transported by ambulance.

3. Alternate Light Source: If community standard, examine patient with Wood's Lamp/ALS.

   — NOTE: Collect specimens from all areas based on history regardless if negative or positive fluorescence PLUS any areas of positive fluorescence.

4. Oral specimens: When history includes oral assault or is unknown for oral assault, consider collecting oral specimens as soon as possible and allowing patient to complete oral hygiene.

   — Collect specimens from lips, around mouth, and corners of mouth.

   — Collect specimens from oral cavity.

   — NOTE: These are NOT buccal swabs for DNA standard. Specimens collected for evidence and buccal swabs for DNA standard are collected from different anatomical locations. Additionally, there should be an oral hygiene protocol between collection of specimens for evidence and collection of buccal swabs for DNA standard. Document oral hygiene in medical forensic record.

5. Collect specimens from both sides of neck.

6. Collect specimens from both breasts.

7. Anogenital specimens:

   — NOTE: Order of specimen collection varies depending on community standards and agency protocols.

   — Collect vulvar specimens.

   — If practice includes use of Toluidine Blue Dye, apply and assess for injury.

   — Insert speculum and collect specimens from vaginal vault and cervical os.

   — NOTE: If used, document use of lubrication on medical forensic record.

   — Collect specimens from perianal skin, anus, and rectum.

   — NOTE: If practice includes use of anoscope, collect specimens from tissue distal to the tip of anoscope; type of lubrication used should be documented in the medical forensic record.

   — If drainage observed from any genital orifice, collect specimen of drainage.

8. Collect blood and toxicology screens per community standard or agency protocol. If history includes concern for drug-facilitated sexual assault, collect blood and urine as soon as possible.

9. DNA standard: Method and time of collection will vary based on community standards and agency protocols.

— If practice is to collect buccal specimens for DNA standard, this may be completed following oral assessment or at the end of the exam if history does not warrant assessment of the oral cavity.

— If practice is to collect blood specimens for DNA standard (eg, blood standard card, tube of blood), this may be completed when other lab specimens are collected; if other lab specimens are not collected during the exam, this may be completed at the end of the exam.

10. If patient must urinate prior to exam, give 4x4 gauze pad to wipe vulva prior to urination and another 4x4 gauze pad to wipe vulva following urination. Collect both 4x4 gauze pads and add these items to the evidence kit.

11. Patient reports ingesting one "beer" and one "shooter"; if law enforcement is involved, inform of concern of drug-facilitated sexual assault and potential evidence on items patient consumed the beer and shooter from.

Activity 5-3. Treatment

— If applicable or desired by patient, offer pregnancy testing and Emergency Hormonal Contraception and provide related patient education.

— Recommend and/or provide medications based on Centers for Disease Control (CDC) guidelines or local/community protocol and provide related patient education.

— Offer STI screenings including HIV screening, referral, and post-exposure prophylaxis (PEP) per CDC guidelines or local/community protocols and provide related patient education.

— Refer for counseling services via rape crisis center, advocacy program, or other local service provider or counseling center.

— Refer to Victim Witness program for assistance with medical expenses not related to the medical forensic examination.

— Provide discharge instructions for care of injury, including a reminder of the presence of Toluidine Blue Dye, and provide anticipatory guidance based on patient history, verbal/nonverbal communication during examination, and patient questions.

Chapter 6: Sexual Assault: 17-year-old Female Patient

Anatomical Skills 6-1

A. Soft palate

B. Left palatopharyngeal arch

C. Left palatoglossal arch

D. Right tonsil

E. Posterior oropharynx

F. Uvula

Activity 6-1. Injury Identification

— Palatoglossal arch: Bilateral generalized redness (**Figure 6-2**)

— Palatopharyngeal arch: Bilateral generalized redness (**Figure 6-2**)

— Uvula: Generalized redness (**Figure 6-2**)

Activity 6-2. Injury Identification

— Posterior fourchette/Fossa navicularis: Posterior fourchette laceration at 6 o'clock extending onto fossa navicularis (**Figure 6-3**)

— Perianal tissue/anus: Circumferential perianal swelling extending onto anal verge and into anal canal; multiple lacerations at 12, 1, 6, 7, and 8 o'clock with active bleeding upon manipulation (**Figure 6-4**)

Activity 6-3. Evidence Collection

1. Photodocumentation: In many communities, photodocumentation will also be used as evidence in the investigative and judicial processes. Photodocumentation should occur throughout the medical forensic examination/evaluation and may include the following:

— Patient upon initial presentation

— Anterior and posterior hands

— Foreign debris or substances on patient or clothing

— Injuries

2. Clothing: Patient ran to neighbor's house naked; collect any items she may have used to cover up with while waiting for the ambulance.

   — Notify law enforcement that original items of clothing are not with patient.

3. Alternate Light Source: If community standard, examine patient with Wood's Lamp/ALS.

   — NOTE: Collect specimens from all areas based on history regardless if negative or positive fluorescence PLUS any areas of positive fluorescence.

4. Oral specimens: When history includes oral assault or is unknown for oral assault, consider collecting oral specimens as soon as possible and allowing patient to complete oral hygiene.

   — Collect specimens from lips, around mouth, and corners of mouth.

   — Collect specimens from oral cavity.

   — NOTE: These are NOT buccal swabs for DNA standard. Specimens collected for evidence and buccal swabs for DNA standard are collected from different anatomical locations. Additionally, there should be an oral hygiene protocol between collection of specimens for evidence and collection of buccal swabs for DNA standard. Document oral hygiene in medical forensic record.

5. Collect specimens from both sides of neck.

6. Collect specimens from both breasts.

7. Anogenital specimens:

   — NOTE: Order of specimen collection varies depending on community standards and agency protocols.

   — Collect vulvar specimens.

   — If practice includes use of Toluidine Blue Dye, apply and assess for injury.

   — Insert speculum and collect specimens from vaginal vault and cervical os.

      — NOTE: If used, document use of lubrication on medical forensic record.

   — Collect specimens from perianal skin, anus, and rectum.

      — NOTE: If practice includes use of anoscope, collect specimens from tissue distal to the tip of anoscope; type of lubrication used should be documented in the medical forensic record.

   — If drainage observed from any genital orifice, collect specimen of drainage.

8. Collect blood and toxicology screens per community standard or agency protocol.

9. DNA standard: Method and time of collection will vary based on community standards and agency protocols.

   — If practice is to collect buccal specimens for DNA standard, this may be completed following oral assessment or at the end of the exam if history does not warrant assessment of the oral cavity.

   — If practice is to collect blood specimens for DNA standard (eg, blood standard card, tube of blood), this may be completed when other lab specimens are collected; if other lab specimens are not collected during the exam, this may be completed at the end of the exam.

10. If patient must urinate prior to exam, give 4x4 gauze pad to wipe vulva prior to urination and another 4x4 gauze pad to wipe vulva following urination. Collect both 4x4 gauze pads and add these items to the evidence kit.

Activity 6-4. Treatment

— Recommend patient see emergency department provider (eg, MD, NP, PA) for evaluation secondary to loss of consciousness.

— If applicable or desired by patient, offer pregnancy testing and Emergency Hormonal Contraception and provide related patient education.

— Recommend and/or provide medications based on Centers for Disease Control (CDC) guidelines or local/community protocol and provide related patient education.

— Offer STI screenings including HIV screening, referral, and post-exposure prophylaxis (PEP) per CDC guidelines or local/community protocols and provide related patient education.

— Refer for counseling services via rape crisis center, advocacy program, or other local service provider or counseling center.

— Refer to Victim Witness program for assistance with medical expenses not related to the medical forensic examination.

— Provide discharge instructions for care of injury, including a reminder of the presence of Toluidine Blue Dye, and provide anticipatory guidance based on patient history, verbal/nonverbal communication during examination, and patient questions.

Chapter 7: Incapacitated Sexual Assault: 24-year-old Female Patient in a Psychiatric Facility

Anatomical Skills 7-1

A. Left labia majora

B. Periurethral bands

C. Hymen

D. Posterior fourchette

E. Perineum

Anatomical Skills 7-2

A. Anus

B. Perianal tissue

C. Anal skin folds

Activity 7-1. Injury Identification

— Vaginal vestibule: Generalized vestibular redness (**Figure 7-3**)

— Fossa navicularis: Abrasion from 4 to 7 o'clock with positive dye uptake (**Figure 7-3**)

— Hymen: Generalized redness (**Figure 7-3**)

— Perianal tissue/anus: Perianal redness from 6 to 7 o'clock; perianal redness and swelling from 9 to 1 o'clock with fecal matter present; laceration at 10 o'clock (**Figure 7-4**)

Activity 7-2. Evidence Collection

1. Photodocumentation: In many communities, photodocumentation will also be used as evidence in the investigative and judicial processes. Photodocumentation should occur throughout the medical forensic examination/evaluation and may include the following:

   — Patient upon initial presentation

   — Anterior and posterior hands

   — Foreign debris or substances on patient or clothing

   — Injuries

2. Clothing: Collect clothing patient was wearing upon arrival.

3. Alternate Light Source: If community standard, examine patient with Wood's Lamp/ALS.
   - — NOTE: Collect specimens from all areas based on history regardless if negative or positive fluorescence PLUS any areas of positive fluorescence.
4. Oral specimens: When history includes oral assault or is unknown for oral assault, consider collecting oral specimens as soon as possible and allowing patient to complete oral hygiene.
   - — Collect specimens from lips, around mouth, and corners of mouth.
   - — Collect specimens from oral cavity.
   - — NOTE: These are NOT buccal swabs for DNA standard. Specimens collected for evidence and buccal swabs for DNA standard are collected from different anatomical locations. Additionally, there should be an oral hygiene protocol between collection of specimens for evidence and collection of buccal swabs for DNA standard. Document oral hygiene in medical forensic record.
5. Collect specimens from both sides of neck.
6. Collect specimens from both breasts.
7. Anogenital specimens:
   - — NOTE: Order of specimen collection varies depending community standards and agency protocols.
   - — Collect vulvar specimens.
   - — If practice includes use of Toluidine Blue Dye, apply and assess for injury.
   - — Insert speculum and collect specimens from vaginal vault and cervical os.
     - — NOTE: If used, document use of lubrication on medical forensic record.
   - — Collect specimens from perianal skin, anus, and rectum.
     - — NOTE: If practice includes use of anoscope, collect specimens from tissue distal to the tip of anoscope; type of lubrication used should be documented in the medical forensic record.
   - — If drainage observed from any genital orifice, collect specimen of drainage.
8. Collect blood and toxicology screens per community standard or agency protocol. History included concern for incapacitated sexual assault, so collect blood and urine as soon as possible.
9. DNA standard: Method and time of collection will vary based on community standards and agency protocols.
   - — If practice is to collect buccal specimens for DNA standard, this may be completed following oral assessment or at the end of the exam if the history does not warrant assessment of the oral cavity.
   - — If practice is to collect blood specimens for DNA standard (eg, blood standard card, tube of blood), this may be completed when other lab specimens are collected; if other lab specimens are not collected during the exam, this may be completed at the end of the exam.
10. If patient must urinate prior to exam, give 4x4 gauze pad to wipe vulva prior to urination and another 4x4 gauze pad to wipe vulva following urination. Collect both 4x4 gauze pads and add these items to the evidence kit.

Activity 7-3. Treatment

- — If applicable or desired by patient, offer pregnancy testing and Emergency Hormonal Contraception and provide related patient education.
- — Recommend and/or provide medications based on Centers for Disease Control (CDC) guidelines or local/community protocol and provide related patient education.
- — Offer STI screenings including HIV screening, referral, and post-exposure prophylaxis (PEP) per CDC guidelines or local/community protocols and provide related patient education.
- — Refer for counseling services via rape crisis center, advocacy program, or other local service provider or counseling center.

— Refer to Victim Witness program for assistance with medical expenses not related to the medical forensic examination.

— Discharge instructions for care of injury, including a reminder of the presence of Toluidine Blue Dye, and provide anticipatory guidance based on patient history, verbal/nonverbal communication during examination, and patient questions.

— NOTE: If patient was not returning to the mental health facility, a social services referral would be appropriate.

Chapter 8: Sexual Assault and Intimate Partner Violence: 32-year-old Female Patient

Anatomical Skills 8-1

A. Mons pubis

B. Clitoral hood

C. Clitoris

D. Left and right labia majora

E. Hymen

Activity 8-1. Injury Identification

— Posterior fourchette: Abrasion extending onto fossa navicularis and multiple lacerations with positive dye uptake (**Figures 8-2** and **8-3**)

— Fossa navicularis: Abrasion with positive dye uptake (**Figures 8-2** and **8-3**)

— Perianal tissue/anus: Lacerations at 1, 4, and 7 o'clock extending onto anal verge with positive dye uptake (**Figure 8-4**)

Activity 8-2. Evidence Collection

1. Photodocumentation: In many communities, photodocumentation will also be used as evidence in the investigative and judicial processes. Photodocumentation should occur throughout the medical forensic examination/evaluation and may include the following:

   — Patient upon initial presentation

   — Anterior and posterior hands

   — Foreign debris or substances on patient or clothing

   — Injuries

2. Clothing: Collect clothing; if applicable, collect second pair of underwear worn.

   — If clothing changed prior to arrival and law enforcement is involved, notify law enforcement that original items of clothing are not with patient.

3. Alternate Light Source: If community standard, examine patient with Wood's Lamp/ALS.

   — NOTE: Collect specimens from all areas based on history regardless if negative or positive fluorescence PLUS any areas of positive fluorescence.

4. Collect specimen from areas patient reports being grabbed (touch DNA).

5. Anogenital specimens:

   — NOTE: The history includes cunnilingus performed on patient AND penetration (vaginal and anorectal) with a foreign object. Specimen collection is based on acts of cunnilingus, however, a speculum exam should still be completed to assess for injury.

   — Collect vulvar specimens.

   — Collect specimens from perianal skin.

— If drainage observed from any genital orifice, collect specimen of drainage.

6. Collect blood and toxicology screens per community standard or agency protocol.
7. DNA standard: Method and time of collection will vary based on community standards and agency protocols.
   — If practice is to collect buccal specimens for DNA standard, this may be completed following oral assessment or at the end of the exam if the history does not warrant assessment of the oral cavity.

   — If practice is to collect blood specimens for DNA standard (eg, blood standard card, tube of blood), this may be completed when other lab specimens are collected; if other lab specimens are not collected during the exam, this may be completed at the end of the exam.
8. If patient must urinate prior to exam, give 4x4 gauze pad to wipe vulva prior to urination and another 4x4 gauze pad to wipe vulva following urination. Collect both 4x4 gauze pads and add these items to the evidence kit.

Activity 8-3. Treatment

— Recommend patient see emergency department provider (eg, MD, NP, PA) for evaluation of increasing abdominal pain.

— Recommend and/or provide medications based on Centers for Disease Control (CDC) guidelines or local/community protocol and provide related patient education.

— Offer STI screenings including HIV screening, referral, and post-exposure prophylaxis (PEP) per CDC guidelines or local/community protocols and provide related patient education.

— NOTE: The nurse acknowledges this is intimate partner violence, however, the options for prophylaxis should still be discussed

— Refer to social work (eg, safety planning, shelter)

— Refer for counseling services via rape crisis center, advocacy program, or other local service provider or counseling center.

— Refer to Victim Witness program for assistance with medical expenses not related to the medical forensic examination.

— Provide discharge instructions for care of injury, including a reminder of the presence of Toluidine Blue Dye, and provide anticipatory guidance based on patient history, verbal/nonverbal communication during examination, and patient questions.

— Discuss follow-up for additional injury documentation if needed (if bruising occurs from restraints).

Chapter 9: Sexual Assault: 20-year-old Female Patient

Anatomical Skills 9-1

A. Left labia minora

B. Hymen

C. Vaginal introitus

D. Fossa navicularis

E. Posterior fourchette

Activity 9-1. Injury Identification

— No injury observed (**Figure 9-2**).

Activity 9-2. Evidence Collection

1. Photodocumentation: In many communities, photodocumentation will also be used as evidence in the investigative and judicial processes. Photodocumentation should occur throughout the medical forensic examination/evaluation and may include the following:
   — Patient upon initial presentation

— Anterior and posterior hands

— Foreign debris or substances on patient or clothing

— Injuries

2. Clothing: Collect clothing patient was wearing upon arrival.
3. Alternate Light Source: If community standard, examine patient with Wood's Lamp/ALS.

   — NOTE: Collect specimens from all areas based on history regardless if negative or positive fluorescence PLUS any areas of positive fluorescence.
4. Collect specimens from both sides of neck (touch DNA).
5. Anogenital specimens:

   — NOTE: Order of specimen collection varies depending on community standards and agency protocols.

   — Collect vulvar specimens.

   — If practice includes use of Toluidine Blue Dye, apply and assess for injury.

   — Insert speculum and collect specimens from vaginal vault and cervical os.

   — NOTE: If used, document use of lubrication on medical forensic record.

   — If drainage observed from any genital orifice, collect specimen of drainage.
6. Collect blood and toxicology screens per community standard or agency protocol. If history includes concern for drug-facilitated sexual assault, collect blood and urine as soon as possible.
7. DNA standard: Method and time of collection will vary based on community standards and agency protocols.

   — If practice is to collect buccal specimens for DNA standard, this may be completed following oral assessment or at the end of the exam if history does not warrant assessment of the oral cavity.

   — If practice is to collect blood specimens for DNA standard (eg, blood standard card, tube of blood), this may be completed when other lab specimens are collected; if other lab specimens are not collected during the exam, this may be completed at the end of the exam.
8. If patient must urinate prior to exam, give 4x4 gauze pad to wipe vulva prior to urination and another 4x4 gauze pad to wipe vulva following urination. Collect both 4x4 gauze pads and add these items to the evidence kit.

Activity 9-3. Treatment

— If applicable or desired by patient, offer pregnancy testing and Emergency Hormonal Contraception and provide related patient education.

— Recommend and/or provide medications based on Centers for Disease Control (CDC) guidelines or local/community protocol and provide related patient education.

— Offer STI screenings including HIV screening, referral, and post-exposure prophylaxis (PEP) per CDC guidelines or local/community protocols and provide related patient education.

— Refer for counseling services via rape crisis center, advocacy program, or other local service provider or counseling center.

— Refer to Victim Witness program for assistance with medical expenses not related to the medical forensic examination.

— Provide anticipatory guidance based on patient history, verbal/nonverbal communication during examination, and patient questions.

Chapter 10: Documenting a History and Reviewing a Case

Injury identification, evidence collection, and treatment will depend on the case chosen by the student, its attendant photographs, and the patient's history.

CME/CNE QUESTIONS

TEST QUESTIONS FOR CHAPTERS 1-10

ENTRY-LEVEL ADOLESCENT AND ADULT SEXUAL ASSAULT ASSESSMENT

ISBN: 978-1-936590-00-1

See pages xiv-xv for submission instructions. If you are unable to submit all required forms through the Saint Louis University CME website, photocopy the posttest, evaluation form, and credits/contact hours form; complete; and return by post or electronic mail.

1. **Superficial injuries representing the removal of the outermost layers of the skin; usually caused by lateral rubbing, sliding, or compressive forces are called:**
   a. Lacerations
   b. Petechiae
   c. Abrasions
   d. Avulsions

2. **The following occurs when the continuity of the skin is broken and disrupted by blunt force such as tearing, ripping, crushing, overstretching, pulling apart, overbending, or shearing of tissue:**
   a. Bruises
   b. Lacerations
   c. Cuts
   d. Abrasions

3. **This is a generic term given to all types of sexual assault when drugs, alcohol, or other intoxicants are deliberately given to the victim by the perpetrator:**
   a. Incapacitated sexual assault
   b. Drug-induced sexual assault
   c. Self-facilitated sexual assault
   d. Drug-facilitated sexual assault

4. **These lie below the intact epidermis and result from extravascular collection of blood that has leaked from ruptured capillaries or blood vessels after sufficient force has been applied to distort the soft tissues and tear one or more vessels:**
   a. Bruises
   b. Petechiae
   c. Contusions
   d. Both a and c

5. **Which of the following is NOT caused by blunt force trauma?**
   a. Cuts
   b. Bruises
   c. Lacerations
   d. Contusions

6. **Which of the following is a small fold of mucous membrane that limits the movement of the tongue?**
   a. Gingiva
   b. Pharynx
   c. Frenum
   d. Uvula

7. **The anterior part of the palate, covered above by the mucous membrane of the nose and below by the mucoperiosteum of the roof of the mouth is known as the:**
   a. Soft palate
   b. Hard palate
   c. Uvular palate
   d. Tonsilar palate

8. **The anterior of 2 folds of mucous membrane on either side of the oropharynx and enclosing related muscles is known as the:**
   a. Uvula
   b. Frenum
   c. Palatopharyngeal arch
   d. Palatoglossal arch

9. **The rounded, prominent border of the glans on the distal portion of the penile shaft is called the:**
   a. Corona of glans penis
   b. Coronal sulcus
   c. Glans
   d. Median raphe

10. **A visible line of tissue extending from the anus to the perineum in both men and women is called the:**
    a. Perineal line
    b. Posterior demarcation
    c. Median raphe
    d. Sulcus of the perineum

11. **The rounded border of the glans penis, separated from the corpora cavernosa penis by the neck of the glans, is called the:**
    a. Coronal sulcus
    b. Corona of glans penis
    c. Scrotum
    d. Glans

12. **The portion of the uterus between the isthmus and the vagina is called the:**
    a. Clitoris
    b. Vaginal rugae
    c. Cervix
    d. Both a and c

13. **A small cylindrical, erectile body at the anterior portion of the vulva is called the:**
    a. Clitoris
    b. Glans
    c. Clitoral hood
    d. Hymen

14. **The concavity of the lower part of the vestibule, posterior and inferior to the hymen corona is called the:**
    a. Posterior fornix
    b. Anterior fornix
    c. Fossa navicularis
    d. Posterior fourchette

15. **The structures that support the urethra and the pelvic floor, usually symmetrical, found in pairs, and attached to the pubic symphysis area are called:**
    a. Periurethral bands
    b. Vestibular bands
    c. Urethral ligaments
    d. All of the above

16. **The posterior fourchette is:**
    a. The area where the two labia majora meet posteriorly
    b. The area where the two labia minora meet posteriorly
    c. The area also known as the fossa navicularis
    d. None of the above

17. **When are vagina rugae not present?**
    a. During the menstrual cycle
    b. When there is no estrogen effect
    c. During pregnancy
    d. When there is no progestin effect

18. **A clinically visible line demarcating nonkeratinized squamous epithellia cells from simple columnar cells in the cervical canal is called the:**
    a. Hart's line
    b. Squamocolumnar junction
    c. Median raphe
    d. Pectinate line

19. **Which of the following is found in both men and women?**
    a. Median raphe
    b. Urethral meatus
    c. Both a and b
    d. None of the above

20. **A cavity containing the openings of the vagina, urethra, and Bartholin's glands is called the:**
    a. Vaginal vault
    b. Perineum
    c. Posterior fornix
    d. Vaginal vestibule

21. **The normal vaginal pH range is:**
    a. 3.8–4.5
    b. 4.5–5.2
    c. 5.2–5.8
    d. 5.8–6.9

22. The terminal part of the large intestine, 3 to 4 cm in length, sensitive to pain, surrounded by sphincter muscles, and without lubricating glands is called the:
   a. Anal verge
   b. Anus
   c. Rectum
   d. Anal canal

23. The pooling of venus blood in the circumferential veins of the anus, marked by a bulging of the veins and flat, purple discoloration of the perianal tissue is called:
   a. Injury
   b. Perianal bruising
   c. Perianal venous engorgement
   d. Both a and b

24. The saw-toothed line of demarcation between the lower portion of the anal verge and the pectin, a smooth zone of stratified squamous epithelium extending to the anal verge is called:
   a. Hart's line
   b. Squamocolumnar junction
   c. Median raphe
   d. Pectinate line

25. Injuries will always be observed during a medical forensic exam of a patient reporting penetration of the vagina or anus or both.
   a. True
   b. False
   c. True if the patient is an adolescent
   d. False if the patient is an adult

www.ingramcontent.com/pod-product-compliance
Lightning Source LLC
LaVergne TN
LVHW070901210926
848482LV00016B/989
9781936590001